# THE FIRST-TIME MOM'S
# BREASTFEEDING HANDBOOK

# THE FIRST-TIME MOM'S

# BREASTFEEDING HANDBOOK

## A MONTH-BY-MONTH GUIDE
### from First Latch
### to Weaning

By Chrisie Rosenthal, IBCLC

Illustrations by Abbie Winters

ROCKRIDGE
PRESS

Series Designer: Julie Schrader
Interior and Cover Designer: Suzanne LaGasa
Art Producer: Hannah Dickerson
Editor: Mo Mozuch
Production Manager: Holly Haydash
Production Editor: Melissa Edeburn
Illustrations © Abbie Winters
Author photo courtesy of Marc Blackwell, Blackwell Studios

ISBN: Print 978-1-64739-950-4 | eBook 978-1-64739-561-2
R0

*This book is dedicated to all the families
and caregivers just starting out on their feeding
journey. Together we've got this!*

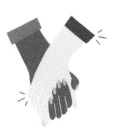

# Contents

## PART THREE: MONTHS 7 TO 12

## PART FOUR: DECIDING WHAT'S NEXT

# Introduction

Hi there! I'm so happy you found this book and that I get to support you on your breastfeeding journey.

Eighteen years ago, after two rounds of IVF, I was pregnant with twin boys and starting *my* mothering journey. At the time I was a producer in the film industry, so creating and executing plans was my forte! I took every class available to me, including Breastfeeding 101 and Preparing for Twins. And then the babies came—and my well-researched plans flew right out the window. Breastfeeding did not start out the way I had envisioned it, and I was never able to get back on track. Although I reached out for lactation support, I didn't get the kind I needed. I combo-fed (used breastmilk and formula) for six months, then formula fed until my boys reached one year.

With my third son, and a little bit of experience under my belt, I was determined to do everything I could to reach my breastfeeding goal. I took all the classes (again!), and I connected with a new lactation consultant during my pregnancy. We put together a game plan, including when and how to get help, to help me reach my goal of breastfeeding for one year. I had lots of issues along the way (plugged ducts, mastitis, low supply, dysphoric milk ejection reflex or D-MER), but I worked through them and had a great experience. I breastfed my youngest son for more than two years because that was what worked best for the two of us.

Two vastly different breastfeeding experiences taught me that the *right support* is essential to meeting your feeding goals. I also learned how important breastfeeding is to the health of our babies. With three little ones under five, I decided to make a career change. I became an IBCLC (lactation consultant) and an advocate for supporting *all* moms on their feeding journey. I'm passionate about providing nonjudgmental breastfeeding support to *all* moms, whether they are breastfeeding exclusively, combo-feeding, pumping exclusively, or weaning (for *whatever* reason).

Over the past 10 years, I've provided inpatient and outpatient breastfeeding support to postpartum families at two large Los Angeles hospitals, supported families in the neonatal intensive care unit (NICU) with premature and compromised babies, taught hospital prenatal breastfeeding 101 classes as well as small group and private feeding classes, worked with pediatric practices, and provided thousands of private lactation consultations through my private practice, The Land of Milk and Mommy. I've also published two books on breastfeeding and provided content and support to families around the world through Cleo, an online platform dedicated to offering support for working parents.

I hope this book empowers you to meet your goals at *every stage* of your feeding journey.

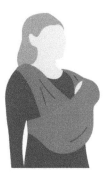

# How to Use This Book

This book is different than other breastfeeding books. It breaks the feeding journey down month by month and week by week, so you can focus on the goal that's right in front of you. You don't need to read this book cover to cover before baby arrives. In fact, I recommend you don't.

"Part One: The Basics" would be most helpful prior to your baby's birth. This section covers the fundamental knowledge you need to get started. (I recommend bookmarking "21 Troubleshooting Tips" on page 42.) Once baby is here, start on "Part Two: Months 1 to 6" (and later "Part Three: Months 7 to 12"). Focus on the challenges and tips for each month (and week).

When it's time, head to "Part Four: Deciding What's Next." It answers your questions about breastfeeding toddlers and guides you through the process of weaning, whether you start the process when your baby is an infant or a toddler.

This book is intended to support *all parents:* same-sex parents, transgender parents, non-binary parents, single parents, adoptive parents, and parents from different ethnic and socioeconomic backgrounds. Whether breastfeeding exclusively, combo-feeding, pumping exclusively, or weaning, parents will find answers to their feeding questions here.

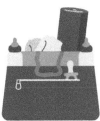

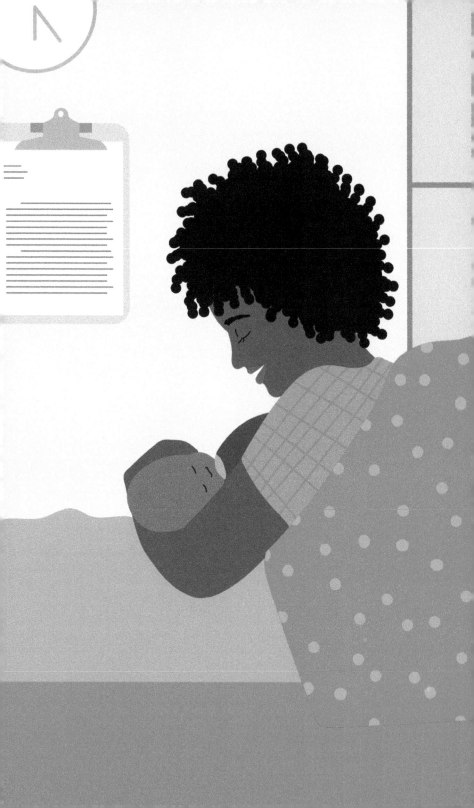

# PART ONE

# The Basics

## Breastfeeding for Beginners

Congratulations on starting your breastfeeding journey! This chapter explains what happens in the body of a pregnant and lactating woman and explores the benefits of breastfeeding for mom and baby. It also offers suggestions on building a support system—from partners, to other moms, to medical professionals—to help you both before and after baby arrives. Finally, it provides a checklist of essential supplies for your breastfeeding journey.

Let's start with the most important piece of advice: **Take feeding one step at a time.** Breastfeeding a newborn is *very different* from breastfeeding a toddler, so try not to worry about the days ahead. Because I want you to take the feeding journey one step at a time, this book breaks it down to weeks and months for easily digestible (pun intended) sections to guide you through the first year.

For most moms, the first few weeks of feeding are the hardest. Good news: Breastfeeding gets *much* easier. YOU CAN DO THIS!

## Biology Basics

Did you know your body started making colostrum (the first breastmilk you produce) around week 14 of your pregnancy? High levels of progesterone in your body during pregnancy keep the milk from increasing and being secreted in significant amounts. (By the way, if you've been leaking colostrum during your pregnancy, that's super normal. And if you haven't, that's super normal too.) You may have noticed your breasts are fuller and more tender in pregnancy. The areola may also become darker and develop pimple-like bumps on or around it called Montgomery's glands. Your breasts are actively undergoing changes to prepare for the task ahead: breastfeeding.

After your baby's birth, the placenta is delivered, which causes a sudden drop in progesterone and estrogen. When those hormones drop and high levels of the hormone prolactin are present, your body knows it's "game on" and begins transitioning to the next stage of breastmilk. You'll see an increase in volume from days three to five, and your breastmilk will shift from colostrum to transitional milk.

Transitional milk is a combination of colostrum and mature milk. This stage lasts for one to two weeks. Your breastmilk contains more colostrum at first, and less and less each day until it's entirely mature milk.

Fun fact: Colostrum and transitional milk are part of the endocrine control system. They happen automatically and are driven by hormones. For the most part, every mom has colostrum and every mom's milk will transition. However, establishing and protecting your mature milk supply is not automatic. *It's all demand and supply.* The more frequently you remove milk from your breasts (and the more milk removed), the more milk you will have. Your supply is always responding to milk removal and can be increased or reduced. Your supply is not "locked in" at any one point in time.

## Why Breastfeed?

Sure, you've heard that breastfeeding is best for babies. But *why* exactly? We'll get to that shortly.

Perhaps *you're* committed to breastfeeding and your partner (or extended family) doesn't understand why it's such a "big deal" to you. It's important to get your partner on board, if possible. Studies show that a partner's support is one of the key factors in determining how long babies are breastfed.

Or, sometimes grandma didn't breastfeed, and she frequently offers to "help out" with a bottle of formula so mom can "take a break," or even questions whether you have enough milk for the baby.

You may be the first in your circle to breastfeed and be missing the support and experience of family or friends who came before you and normalized breastfeeding.

All these situations are challenging. The more information you have, the better prepared you are to have conversations about the benefits of breastfeeding, so you can feel supported in achieving your goal.

There are also many breastfeeding benefits for mom too—and this topic doesn't get nearly enough attention.

So, let's take a look at what we know, and why breastfeeding is the golden standard for feeding your baby.

## BENEFITS FOR BABY

The list is long, but some of the many health benefits of breastfeeding include lowering your baby's risk of allergies, bacterial meningitis, childhood leukemia, diabetes, diarrhea, obesity, respiratory infections, SIDS, ear infections, and inflammatory bowel disease.

Breastmilk is also nature's own immunity booster. Because breastmilk contains huge numbers of antibodies, babies who breastfeed are less likely to get sick. According to the American Academy of Pediatrics, human milk "contains many substances that benefit your baby's immune system, including antibodies, immune factors, enzymes, and white blood cells. These substances protect your baby against a wide variety of diseases and infections not only while he is breastfeeding but, in some cases, long after he has weaned. Formula cannot offer this protection." Cool fact: When you breastfeed, your body takes in germs from your baby's mouth and skin and makes antibodies specific to your baby's environment. Pretty amazing, right?

We're also learning that the mechanics of breastfeeding may lend specific benefits to the development of the breastfed baby's jaw, dental health, and airway. Babies have to work harder at breastfeeding (versus bottle-feeding) and use their mouths in a completely different way. This may factor into lower rates of SIDS and lead to less tooth crowding and better jaw alignment.

## BENEFITS FOR MOM

Breastfeeding has important benefits for mom too. Research tells us that breastfeeding helps protect mothers even after weaning by lowering the risks of breast cancer, heart disease, high blood pressure, high cholesterol, ovarian cancer, rheumatoid arthritis, and type 2 diabetes.

When it comes to breast and ovarian cancers, research is showing that the more time a mom spends breastfeeding, the lower her risk. Women who breastfeed for more than 12 months in their lifetime have a 28 percent lower risk of breast cancer, and for women who ever breastfed, a 22 percent lower risk of ovarian cancer.

Research also shows that oxytocin (released during breast-feeding) helps reduce postpartum bleeding by promoting more frequent and intense uterine contractions and facilitating faster uterine involution (the uterus returning to its previous smaller size). That's a significant and important health benefit!

Breastfeeding typically delays a mom's menstrual period for many months and helps space children naturally. The effect is so strong it's used as a family planning method, called the lactational amenorrhea method (LAM). If followed perfectly in the first six months, LAM is about 98 percent effective. (To use this method, you must give your baby only breastmilk and breastfeed every four hours during the day and every six hours at night. This regimen keeps your body from ovulating and prevents you from getting pregnant.)

Breastfeeding hormones—especially oxytocin, known as the "love hormone"—promote bonding with baby and help mom feel relaxed. When your baby latches and starts feeding, your pituitary gland floods your brain with oxytocin, typically bringing feelings of relaxation, safety, and bliss. Your baby's body also releases oxytocin while breastfeeding. This is nature reinforcing the breastfeeding behavior, facilitating mutual bonding, and encouraging both of you to keep doing what you're doing.

Because breastfeeding burns an extra 200 to 500 calories per day, many moms find losing weight easier while breastfeeding. If you want to actively work on weight loss, wait until month two at a minimum and aim to keep weight loss under 1.5 pounds a week. More rapid weight loss could affect your milk supply.

Breastfeeding is also much less expensive than formula and is more convenient. (Breastmilk is always there and ready to go!) Some estimates put formula feeding at more than $1,500 per year.

Last but not least, studies show that breastfeeding parents get more sleep at night. One study found that women who exclusively breastfeed at night averaged 30 minutes more of nocturnal sleep compared with those who gave formula at night. And who doesn't want more sleep?

## A Healthy Head Start

The American Academy of Pediatrics is clear about the benefits of breastmilk and its impact on baby's first year:

> Human milk is species-specific, and all substitute feeding preparations differ markedly from it, making human milk uniquely superior for infant feeding. Exclusive breastfeeding is the reference or normative model against which all alternative feeding methods must be measured with regard to growth, health, development, and all other short- and long-term outcomes. In addition, human milk-fed premature

infants receive significant benefits with respect to host protection and improved developmental outcomes compared with formula-fed premature infants ... pediatricians and parents should be aware that exclusive breastfeeding is sufficient to support optimal growth and development for approximately the first six months of life and provides continuing protection against diarrhea and respiratory tract infection. Breastfeeding should be continued for at least the first year of life and beyond for as long as mutually desired by mother and child.

The World Health Organization and UNICEF say, "exclusive breastfeeding for the first six months of life is the recommended way of feeding infants, followed by continued breastfeeding with appropriate complementary foods for **up to two years or beyond**."

Trust the experts. Breastfeeding gives your child the best start in life and is the perfect nutrition for your baby.

Unfortunately, as you may have experienced, breastfeeding remains a struggle for many women. According to a CDC study of infants born in the United States in 2015, four out of five women started out breastfeeding, but by three months, only half continued.

I hope this isn't your story. May this book be a resource to help you ultimately reach your breastfeeding goal by building your knowledge and troubleshooting any issues that arise.

## Establish Your Support System Early

You shouldn't be in this alone. Think about it: For centuries, we lived together in communities and supported one another through pregnancy, birth, and breastfeeding. Find your village. Build your support network.

The best time to assemble your support team is before baby is here (but don't worry if you didn't get a chance; lots of new moms are in the same boat). Each person below lends a different type of support, and one doesn't take the place of another. Think TEAM. Let's take a look at the places where you can find the people who will be invaluable in your breastfeeding journey.

## YOUR PARTNER

Your partner might be your child's other parent, or if you're single, it might be someone who is dedicated to being on this journey with you. This is your main go-to person who will ideally come to classes with you during your pregnancy, talk with you about parenting styles, and help you do the legwork of physically getting ready for your little one.

This person should be your second set of ears and pair of hands. They are your "tag-team person" when one of you needs a break.

A common misperception is that the partner can't help with breastfeeding. Not true at all! Here are a few ways partners can be involved with breastfeeding:

- Attend a prenatal breastfeeding class with you. Ask questions. Take notes.

- Do research on breast pumps. Order the pump. Assemble the pump.

- Be present for lactation consultations. Be an active participant in troubleshooting and assisting with feeding issues.

- Learn paced bottle-feeding (see "Paced Bottle-Feeding" on page 40).
- Wash and prepare bottle and pump parts.
- Order and be in charge of replacing the silicone pump parts each month.
- Burp baby after breastfeeding or bottle-feeding.
- Tag-team night feeds with mom so you can both get a stretch of sleep.

## YOUR MOM FRIENDS

Mom friends play a special role on your team. They may be your trusted advisors if they have breastfeeding experience. They may be the ones to swing by with food for you or pop in to do a load of laundry or your dishes in those first few crazy weeks. Or they may be the person you text at 2 a.m. when you're both wide awake feeding (again). Either way, these friends are invaluable.

Be honest and let your friends know what you think you'll need. Don't be afraid to ask them how they can help. Try keeping a running "help me" list so when a friend reaches out, you don't have to rack your brain trying to think of what you need at that moment. Ask your mom friends what they would have found helpful when they had newborns and when they were breastfeeding. Tap into that vast knowledge and accept their help. One day you'll be on the other end and be able to pay it forward.

## MOM GROUPS ONLINE

Another great place to connect with moms is online. Finding lots of groups out there is pretty easy. Local breastfeeding moms? Check. Baby-wearing moms? Check. Fitness moms? Check.

Exclusively pumping moms? Check. Moms due the same month as you? Check. Join multiple groups across your social media. See where you fit in. If you aren't feeling it with the groups you've found, start your own.

A nice thing about online groups is you get a cross section of experience, from moms who've dealt with the struggles you're facing to moms in the same boat as you. With a large online group, someone's going to be awake in those early hours when you are. Having a group to reach out to, regardless of the hour, is a huge asset.

## YOUR PEDIATRICIAN

Your pediatrician is an extremely important part of your support network. It's worth putting in the time and research to find a pediatrician you really connect with. When you think about it, this could be your child's doctor for the next 18 years.

Ask your friends and mom groups online for recommendations. Meet several doctors from different practices, make sure you feel comfortable with them, and get a feel for their office and staff. Do you want to be with a big practice, or is a small practice more your style? Do they take your insurance? Are you okay seeing another doctor in the practice if it means getting you in faster? What does their weekend and after-hours coverage look like? Are you on the same page with issues like vaccinations and breastfeeding?

Putting in the time and effort to find the right fit now will pay off greatly down the road.

## LACTATION PROFESSIONAL

Finding an experienced International Board Certified Lactation Consultant (IBCLC, or LC for short) you connect with while pregnant will give you a huge head start. Your IBCLC should be experienced and have positive reviews from other moms in your community. More important, though, you should feel like you understand each other and communicate well. Once you are working together, the LC should make you feel heard, provide education, *plus* develop an actionable plan of care. They should also provide a follow-up period where you can ask questions or modify your plan if needed.

Maybe you liked the LC who taught your prenatal breastfeeding class. Or maybe you have a friend who raves about the LC she used. Your hospital may have LCs available as an outpatient resource or you may find a great LC who is running a breastfeeding support group in your neighborhood.

Wherever you find the LC, connect with them before baby is here so you have that contact in your back pocket. You may not end up needing a breastfeeding consultation, but you'll have the phone number *just in case* you do.

Another convenient way of meeting with LCs, which is becoming more and more common, is the *virtual* lactation consultation. These are online appointments where you may or may not be feeding the baby, but you will have an opportunity to discuss feeding struggles and will leave with a plan of care.

Did you know that under the Affordable Care Act your medical insurance will typically cover (or reimburse for) LCs? This even includes a prenatal consultation. Reach out to an LC familiar with insurance coverage and find out how that works ahead of time.

# The Big Breastfeeding Checklist

It's hard to know exactly what breastfeeding supplies you'll need to have on hand. To make matters worse, when you're pregnant you're bombarded with ads telling you every product is "essential." They're not. To help, I've compiled a checklist to make shopping easier. Many of these items can be borrowed, so check in with friends and family who recently had babies and may not be using these anymore.

**Baby Carrier or Wrap:** A soft wrap or carrier (think one long strip of fabric) or a ring sling are the best choices for the first three months. After month three, you'll also want a structured (backpack-style) carrier, especially for outings. You can practice using the carrier before baby arrives by using a teddy bear or soft doll. Your support people can also do some baby-wearing. Wearing your baby tends to make baby happy and you mobile.

**Bottles:** Get a few bottle brands and make sure you get the slowest flow nipple available. Babies are sometimes the ones to choose the bottle that best works for them. In general, LCs tend to prefer bottles with longer, narrow nipples that mimic the shape and placement of your breast within the baby's mouth. Also, for breastmilk you won't ever need bottles larger than 4 ounces. Your baby's average daily intake plateaus around three weeks at 25 ounces, meaning the average bottle from four weeks on would be 3 to 4 ounces.

**Breastfeeding Pillow:** A great breastfeeding pillow will help you get a good latch in the first few weeks. There are big differences among them, though. Look for a wide base that goes completely around you and snaps together on the side. You want to be sure you choose one that stays in place in order to fully support you and baby.

When you're breastfeeding, the pillow should be right under your breasts, not down at your waist. If it's too low, you'll need to lean over to bring your breast to baby, which will lead to pain in your back and shoulders. If you need to, insert a bed pillow between the feeding pillow and your lap to fill the space.

**Breastfeeding Tank or Shirts:** Wearing the right clothes makes public breastfeeding much easier. Think easy access to your breasts while maintaining coverage. Shirts that button up the front are good options or layer up (such as with a nursing tank under a sweater or bigger shirt).

**Breastmilk Storage Bags:** A popular way of preserving expressed milk in the freezer is with breastmilk storage bags. Some parents like to store in the refrigerator first and move to the freezer after three to four days. Others go straight to the freezer. Either way is fine. Frozen breastmilk is good for approximately six months. Pro tip: Lay the bags flat in the freezer to take up less space.

**Double-Electric Breast Pump:** This is one item you shouldn't need to borrow because your medical insurance company should provide one for you. Give them a call early to learn more about your breastfeeding benefits because many insurers require a prescription for equipment. There is a huge difference in quality between the many double-electric pumps on the market, too, so do your research.

If your medical insurance company only provides one brand (and it's not the one you want), there may be ways around that. Go directly to the manufacturer's website and look through their resources on how to order it. Additionally, many online durable medical equipment (DME) companies will take your medical insurance information, do the legwork, and send you the pump you want. Sometimes it can be more expensive to go through a DME, so explore all your options. Try to have the pump set up before baby arrives. Taking care of it in advance is one less thing to handle when you're home with baby.

**Footstool:** A breastfeeding footstool wins the award for "most often overlooked tool." Using a footstool changes the angle of your thighs so they aren't slanted down, creating a big gap between your breasts and lap. Having your feet raised will make breastfeeding much more ergonomic and easier on your body.

**Hand Pump:** Hand pumps are pretty affordable and everyone should have one. This is the pump you throw in your bag for an emergency. You may also use it for quick "comfort pumps" when your breasts feel full or if you get a plugged duct. It's also "handy" (see what I did there?) when you're in the car or on an airplane and don't have access to an outlet and pumping station.

**Hands-free Pumping Bra:** A hands-free pumping bra is useful whether you're a once-a-day pumper or you're exclusively pumping. It holds the flanges (breast shields) in place, freeing your hands to do other things. Look for one that has Velcro in the back so you can pull it tighter as your body changes over time.

**Hydrogels:** Hydrogels are thin layers of gel to apply to sore nipples. Most moms say they feel even better cold, so try storing them in the refrigerator.

**Nipple Creams or Lanolin:** The best nipple healing product is your own breastmilk. (Simply express a drop and dab.) But many moms also find creams and lanolin soothing. Warning: If you're allergic to wool, you can't use lanolin. To check for an allergic reaction to any product, apply a test spot to the underside or soft part of your arm first and watch for any skin irritation or changes before applying to your nipples.

**Nursing Bra:** You'll definitely want to invest in a good nursing bra. Purchase it two weeks after baby's birth so you'll know what size your breasts will be. If possible, find a store or breastfeeding boutique to size you before you buy anything.

**Nursing Pads:** Some moms leak breastmilk for a few weeks, and some don't. It's a good idea to have some nursing pads on hand just in case. If you find yourself wearing them every day, consider getting them in reusable cloth or bamboo, which is better for the environment and reduces your exposure to chemicals.

**Pacifier:** There are many pacifiers out there. Look for a long and narrow one to replicate the shape and position of your nipple during breastfeeding. When baby is a newborn, you may need to put your finger inside the hollow area of the pacifier and hold it in their mouth. They will get the hang of it over time.

**Silicone "Hand Pump":** These nifty devices attach to the other breast while you're breastfeeding. Contrary to the name, they do not involve actively "pumping." Instead, you squeeze the bulb and attach the flange to your breast. The suction is what removes milk. The hand pump is a HUGE timesaver and a really easy way to start collecting a little extra milk in the first few weeks. Word of warning: Don't overuse. Milk removal is the main way your body establishes your milk supply. If you use it too much, you may push yourself into oversupply. (Oversupply doesn't sound like a problem, but it is.) For most moms, once or twice a day doesn't cause a problem.

# FORMULA AND COMBO-FEEDING

Some families find that breastfeeding exclusively, giving only breast-milk, or feeding at the breast doesn't work out. Although I hope this book will help you navigate your breastfeeding journey, **you shouldn't feel like a failure if breastfeeding doesn't go the way you had pictured it.**

Some decide to combo-feed (breastmilk and formula) or start out breastfeeding and move to formula later. Others prefer not to put the baby to breast, opting instead for pumping and feeding exclusively with bottles ("exclusive pumping").

What's the minimum amount of breastmilk your baby should receive each day to get the benefits? The answer is dose-dependent—the more breastmilk your baby takes in over time, the more benefits they will get. Some breastmilk is better than no breastmilk.

Many families use donated milk or purchase breastmilk from milk banks. All these choices are valid. There's no room for shaming or guilt. *Do what's right for you and your family!*

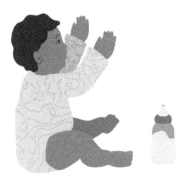

# Latching, Positions, and Supply

Now that you have a bit of background information on your body and baby, let's look at establishing a breastfeeding routine. Your baby will need to be fed a minimum of 8 to 12 times every 24 hours. Having a good routine will help you and baby roll smoothly throughout the day.

An example feeding routine that works for many is breastfeed, burp, change diaper, baby-wear (while you grab a snack or meal), and nap. This chapter covers latching, breastfeeding positions, managing pain and discomfort, and reading baby's cues to make sure they're getting enough. These skills are the foundation for the breastfeeding routine you develop.

## How You'll Know Baby Is Hungry

Breastfeeding starts with a hungry baby. But babies don't just nurse when they're hungry. They may turn to the breast when they're upset, need connection, feel uncomfortable, or are ready to fall asleep (which is called "non-nutritive" or "comfort" nursing). You can tell your baby is hungry when they start exhibiting "hunger cues."

Early signs of hunger, a.k.a. "hunger cues," include:

- Rooting (turning head from side to side)
- Putting hands in their mouth
- Bobbing their head on your chest
- Furrowing their brow or looking irritated
- Throwing their head down toward your breast

**Tip:** Try to catch your baby at the first signs of hunger rather than waiting until they are crying. A mad, crying baby is a frustrated baby, and in that state, they are less likely to open their mouth wide and get a good latch. (On the other hand, you don't always have a choice. Your baby might take a long nap and wake up "hangry." If that happens, let them suck on your finger or a pacifier to calm down, which will give you both a chance to "reset.")

# How You'll Know Baby Is Full

Unless your baby is in a growth spurt (a.k.a. "barracuda baby time"), you'll know when they are full after a feed because they'll seem relaxed and content—possibly even sleepy. Here are some signs to look for to know your baby is done with the feed:

+ Long pauses (more than three seconds) between bursts of sucking
+ Baby appears happy and satiated
+ Hands and body appear relatively limp and relaxed

You may hear you should wait until baby falls asleep or unlatches. Although these events are signs your baby is full, you shouldn't necessarily wait until they occur. Most babies are happy to stay on the breast long after the feed is done.

# Latching

The critical element of a comfortable and effective breastfeed is getting a good latch. Most moms need practice and attention to learn the technique in the beginning, but it becomes second nature over time. This section looks at why the latch is so important, reviews basic latching principles, and provides tips to help you and baby get the hang of this important skill.

### WHAT IS THE LATCH?

"Latching" is the process of your baby attaching to the breast to transfer breastmilk.

It surprises some moms to learn that the baby should be latched *deeply on breast tissue*. A "shallow latch" is when the baby doesn't have enough breast tissue in their mouth and isn't on deep enough. A shallow latch is usually very painful for mom, isn't optimal for milk transfer, and causes very sore nipples over time. A deep latch is always our goal.

## HOW TO GET A GOOD LATCH

Because latching is so important, the pressure on first-time moms to quickly get it right can be intense. Latching takes time to master. Catching your baby's hunger cues as early as possible is key. Try to be patient. *If the latch isn't right, break the latch and start again.* The more you and baby practice, the better you'll get, and pretty soon you'll both be latching pros!

## DEEP LATCH TECHNIQUE

**Hold your baby tummy-to-tummy with you, so their tummy is touching your tummy.** Baby should not be lying on their back with their head turned toward you.

**Line up your nipple with baby's nose.** This tells you you're in the right place to start.

**Express a drop of breastmilk on your nipple.**

**Compress your breast into a "sandwich."** Your fingers should be at least one inch back from the nipple (see "The Breast Sandwich" on page 23).

**Run your nipple over baby's nose and lips and encourage them to open their mouth wide.** You can't get a deep latch unless you get a *big, open wide* mouth first.

**Look for baby to drop their head back as they open wide.**

**Catch your baby's bottom lip first, then their top lip.** It's a one-two motion. Bottom lip first, then top lip, folding in *as much* breast tissue as possible. Your nipple should land at the very back of your baby's hard palate (roof of their mouth), and you should have at least an inch of your breast tissue in your baby's mouth. The more, the better.

**Allow baby's nose and chin to lightly touch your breast as baby feeds.** Don't worry; baby can breathe. They are born with wide noses and recessed chins for breastfeeding. Making an "air pocket" (using your finger to push in the area of your breast closest to baby's nose) moves your nipple inside baby's mouth, which changes your latch and damages your nipple.

## SIGNS OF A GOOD LATCH

How do you know you've got a good latch?

Look for these signs:

- Baby has *at least* an inch of your breast in their mouth.
- Their nose and chin are lightly touching your breast.
- Their lips are curled outward like "fish lips."
- The latch isn't painful (although a little tenderness is normal for the first few weeks).
- Baby is in a suck-swallow-breath pattern, with one to three sucks per swallow.
- You may see motion near the baby's ears.
- You may hear baby swallowing.

Getting a good latch takes practice, but it's worth it. It's the first big skill you and your baby will master together. Once you've got the latch down, the rest is really fine tuning.

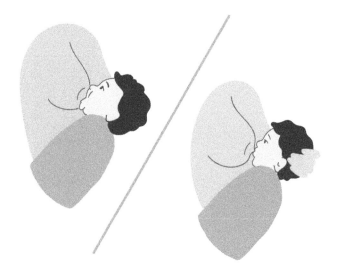

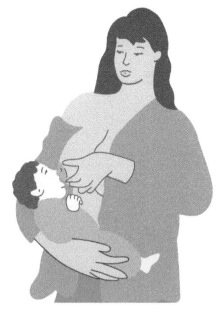

## THE BREAST SANDWICH

"Sandwiching" the breast is key during latching because it helps your baby get as much breast tissue as possible in their mouth. Remember, babies should be latching onto the breast tissue, not the nipple itself. This is why we compress, or gently squeeze, the tissue together.

First, make sure your fingers are at least one inch back from the nipple. You've only got one try, and if your fingers are too close to the nipple, your baby will get stopped there and won't have a chance to latch deeply.

Second, as you compress your breast, your fingers should be opposite each other on the side of your breast. Whether you come in as a "U"- or "C"-shape depends on the position of your baby. You want to match the shape of your baby's mouth. For example, if your baby is in a horizontal position (see "Cross-Cradle Hold" on page 27), you should come in from below your breast and hold your hand in a "U" shape, like you're holding a sandwich.

When baby is latched correctly, their head, shoulders, and hips should be in alignment.

## TONGUE-TIED

You're doing everything "right," and yet the latch is still super painful and your nipples are crazy damaged. Baby seems frustrated, and it's just. not. working. What's going on?

Sometimes the culprit is a tongue-tie. This is when the baby's frenulum (tissue under the tongue) is tight, preventing the tongue from extending beyond the gumline, up to the roof of the mouth, or both. An ear, nose, throat (ENT) doctor or pediatric dentist who has received training in tongue-ties can evaluate and diagnose your baby. If appropriate, they may suggest a "release" or a quick outpatient procedure using a laser or scissors to make a small cut under the baby's tongue. After the procedure, your baby should have full range of motion.

Signs your baby has a tongue-tie:

+ The latch is painful despite getting a deep latch.
+ Baby's weight gain is slow or not meeting expectations.
+ Baby comes off the breast repeatedly and is unable to sustain a latch.
+ After feeding, your nipple comes out of baby's mouth in a "lipstick" shape, where the end is slanted.
+ Milk supply is slow to establish and difficult to maintain.
+ Mom has recurrent plugged ducts.
+ Baby has "reflux" symptoms.

Keep in mind, though, that there are many potential causes for these signs and they don't necessarily mean there's a tongue-tie. Rule out the basics of latch positioning first by using the principles in this book, and consult with the ENT or pediatric dentist. Be aware that some pediatricians are concerned that tongue-ties are being overdiagnosed. If in doubt, a second opinion is always a good idea.

## Assume the Position

So, you found a breastfeeding position you like, and you and baby have settled into a lovely, predictable routine. Suddenly, your baby hits a growth spurt and your nipples are sore. (Ouch!) The thought of putting baby back to breast in the same position is causing you to cringe. Now let's switch it up. Having the ability to vary breastfeeding positions can give you some nipple relief, may allow you to get more comfortable, and gives you flexibility when you find yourself feeding in different locations.

Latching and positioning go hand in hand. There are many different breastfeeding positions or "holds" you can use for feeding your baby. This section will give you instructions on how to use various positions.

There's not necessarily a "right" or "wrong" here. Start with the basics, then experiment. You'll come to find out what feels most comfortable for you and for your baby.

### AUSTRALIAN HOLD

The Australian (or "upright" position) is great for an older baby who has good back and neck strength. In this position, baby is sitting upright on your lap and feeding at the breast. Typically, babies aren't developmentally ready to feed in this position until they are about six months old.

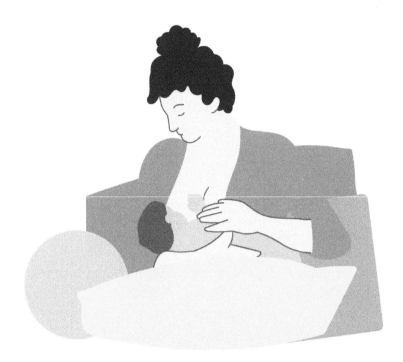

**CRADLE HOLD**

In cradle hold, the baby is positioned horizontally across mom's torso with their head resting in the crook of mom's arm. Mom's other arm is completely free. A cross-cradle hold (see "Cross-Cradle Hold" on page 27) is a typical starting position. Once baby is latched, transition to the cradle hold, which many find much more natural and relaxing.

This position is a mom staple and is great once you have observed that your baby can get *and sustain* a deep latch (typically after week two). Be careful: If you move to the cradle position too early, your baby will move from a deep latch to a shallow latch and your nipples will get very sore.

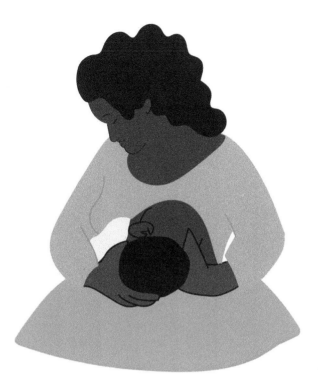

## CROSS-CRADLE HOLD

Begin the cross-cradle hold by sandwiching your breast with the hand closest to your breast. Your other hand holds baby in latching position—tummy to tummy with mom and lined up nose to nipple—securing them firmly behind their ears, neck, and back. Once you latch baby, maintain this position.

It usually takes babies a couple of weeks to learn how to sustain a latch, so in this position you're helping your baby keep that deep latch by holding both "pieces of the puzzle"—baby and breast.

An advantage to the cross-cradle hold is it helps prevent sore nipples. If you started in this position, moved to cradle hold, then experienced sore nipples, return to cross-cradle. Baby may not have mastered sustaining a deep latch. Give them time—they'll get it.

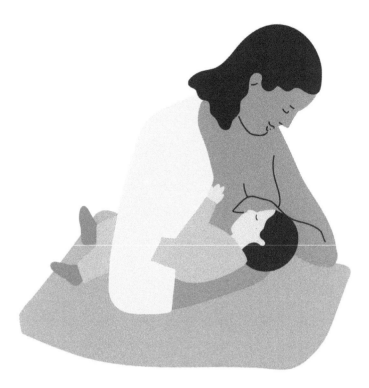

## FOOTBALL OR CLUTCH HOLD

Football (or "clutch") position is when your baby is latched on the breast and their body wraps around the side of your body. In this position, your hand closest to the baby is supporting them behind the ears, neck, and back. Your other hand may be sandwiching your breast or it may be free to do other things if baby can sustain a deep latch. Don't forget to rotate the breastfeeding pillow to the side, so your baby is still fully supported without your body needing to do the work.

The football hold is another great "starter" position, though it can be used any time. This position offers the advantage of allowing you, nurses, LCs, or other support people to get a good view of your baby's latch. It also gets baby off your torso, an added bonus if you're recovering from a cesarean birth.

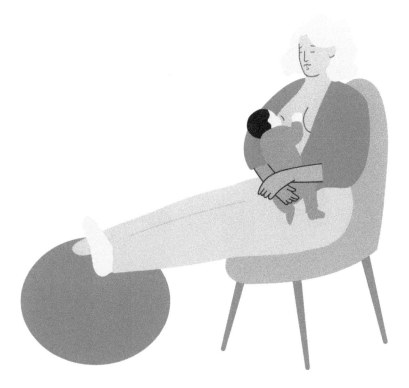

## LAID-BACK HOLD

The laid-back hold is done semi-reclined. In this position, you are leaning back (45 degrees or more) and baby is lying diagonally across your torso. Your arm (the one closest to the breast baby is feeding from) cradles the baby and creates a "nest," your hand supporting baby's bottom. Your back and neck should be supported (try using cushions and pillows while reclining in bed or on a sofa). Babies will typically self-latch in this position.

Also called "biological nurturing," this position is very ergonomic and comfortable for many. It gets you off the perineum and can be great if you had a tear or episiotomy, or are sore from vaginal birth.

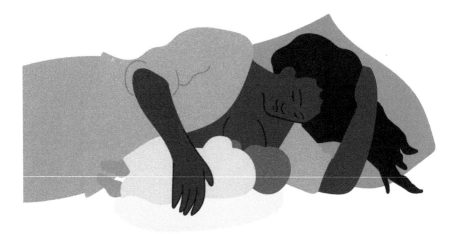

## SIDE-LYING HOLD

Side-lying is another great position to try once your baby is a couple of weeks old and getting the hang of latching. Here, you are lying in bed on your side, tummy to tummy with your baby. Your baby's head is lined up with the breast closest to the bed. You'll have one arm bent, above your head, and the other free to help your baby latch on.

When first learning this position, you may want to roll a blanket into a bolster and tuck it behind your baby's back to keep them on their side and in the correct position.

This is a great position for "nursing down" (getting your baby to feed and fall asleep). It's also super relaxing for you. In fact, you might be able to catch a few zzz's with your baby. Reminder: Always follow the safe sleep rules if you are sharing a space to rest with your baby. A good source to go to if you're unsure of the best way to lie down with baby is *Sweet Sleep: Nighttime and Naptime Strategies for the Breastfeeding Family* (see References, page 165).

# How You'll Know If Baby Is Getting Enough to Eat

Here's the million-dollar question: Now that you can spot a hungry baby and feed them, how do you know they're getting enough breastmilk? With a bottle, you can *see* how many ounces baby ate. It's not the same with the breast. But the good news is there are lots of cues that indicate baby is getting enough.

**Weight Gain:** Weight gain is the *bottom line*. We expect a baby to lose between approximately five and seven percent of their birth weight in the first three to four days of life. They should be back to birth weight by approximately day 14. Then babies are expected to gain 5.5 to 8 ounces per week from ages zero to four months, 3.25 to 4.5 ounces per week from three to six months, and 1.75 to 2.75 ounces per week from six months to one year. If your baby is gaining the appropriate amount of weight, what you are doing is working.

**Output:** In the first few days, output (yes, pees and poops) is watched closely and tells a lot. You and your team will be looking for:

+ Day one: one wet diaper

+ Day two: two wet diapers

+ Day three: three wet diapers

+ Day four and later: six or more wet diapers

+ Stools: Stools should be mustard colored by day five, and at that point, baby should be getting three to four (or more) stools per day. A stool is anything the size of a quarter or larger.

**Visual or Audio Cues at the End of a Feed:** Baby started with an active suck or swallow pattern and gradually transitioned to a slower pattern with three-or-more-second pauses between bursts of sucking; breastfeed took around 15 to 25 minutes (might be faster for moms with a very strong supply); breast is softer after a feed; you may hear swallows; and baby seems satiated and happy.

## Supply

You settle in to breastfeed your baby, and instead of a happy, full baby at the end of the feed, your little one is super upset and acting like they are still very hungry. What happened? Did you suddenly lose all your milk? Is that even possible?

Breastmilk supply is another source of worry for many moms. Often, though, low supply concerns are the result of *perceived* low supply. Most breastfeeding moms have enough milk to feed their baby. And if a mom is not making enough, it's helpful to know supply is always responsive and learn ways to increase it.

Let's look at how supply changes over the first two weeks after birth and what moms can do to help manage how much milk they produce.

### THE FIRST TWO WEEKS

The first two weeks of a first-time mom's breastfeeding journey are the most eventful. For the first three to five days after birth, you'll have colostrum, a highly concentrated, specialized breast-milk. A full serving of colostrum is five to seven milliliters, which matches your baby's tiny tummy size at birth. Colostrum does several magical things: It's high in protein, helps stabilize baby's blood sugar, contains a laxative to help baby move meconium (their first poop), and helps seal your baby's gastrointestinal tract to be less permeable to infection *for life*. (Impressive, right?)

Around days three to five, your milk will increase in volume, and for the next one to two weeks you'll have "transitional milk." This process is automatic and triggered by the delivery of your placenta. At this point, your baby's tummy has grown and is able to comfortably hold about one ounce. By the end of week one, your baby's tummy can comfortably hold up to two ounces. It's the only time in our lives our stomachs grow that fast. What's happening is baby's tummy growth is actually mirroring the stages of mom's milk production.

Your body will also go through three distinct "milk regulations" at two weeks, six weeks, and three months, triggered by hormonal shifts that naturally occur at these times. Your body will be extra sensitive to the messages you're sending regarding how much milk your baby removes and will adjust supply in response.

The following tips for the first two weeks will help ensure your body establishes and sustains appropriate breastmilk production:

### Feed frequently

The primary factor that determines milk supply is the number of times you remove milk from your breasts in a 24-hour period. Your body is expecting a minimum of 8 to 12 feeds every 24 hours. Newborns, as well as babies in growth spurts, usually eat 10 to 12 times every day; otherwise, approximately 8 times a day will be the norm.

### Massage your breasts

Another important factor in establishing and protecting your milk supply is effective milk removal. Breast massage or compressions while breastfeeding will make milk removal much more efficient and speed up feeding time. Use the side of your hand to massage from the top of your breast (by your chest wall) to about hallway down. You don't want to get too close to baby's mouth, though, because that could affect the latch.

### Feed or pump during the night

If you have a partner or support person offering to bottle-feed at night, it's *super* tempting to let them jump in to get a long stretch of restorative sleep. (I get it!) However, doing so can send a signal to your body to reduce milk supply. A good rule of thumb is not to go longer than six hours without feeding or pumping at night during the first six weeks. And this is assuming your breast comfort allows you to go that long. If you're "tag-teaming" with your partner and your breasts are uncomfortable, you'll need to wake up and pump, or you could end up with plugged ducts or mastitis.

### Pump if supplementing

Sometimes bottles and supplementation are necessary. If your goal is to establish a full milk supply, pump both breasts for 15 minutes for each full bottle that's given to your baby to tell your body a feed happened. If you're in the hospital and your pediatrician has asked you to supplement, request a hospital-grade breast pump for your room. You can start pumping right away and use the milk you express to supplement.

### Don't overstimulate

Just like low supply, oversupply is also a problem. Some moms start having issues when they insert extra pump sessions in the first few weeks. It's exciting to start creating a little extra "stash," but you want to be careful you don't send your body the wrong message. Signs of oversupply include having often uncomfortably full breasts, plugged ducts, or mastitis, and a flow that is difficult for baby to control.

## What Affects Your Supply

Many factors drive your milk supply, with frequency and efficacy of milk removal at the top of the list. When you breastfeed, you're removing a small whey protein called Feedback Inhibitor of Lactation (FIL), which sends important signals to your body to make more milk. And, the more milk you remove and the more efficiently you remove it, the more milk you make. In addition to protein removal, the hormone prolactin also assists in the milk synthesis process.

Let's look at risk factors for low supply as well as tips and techniques to increase output.

### HOW MUCH IS NOT ENOUGH?

Your baby is not getting enough if your pediatrician has determined they are not gaining weight appropriately. If you're worried about your breastmilk supply, look at your baby's weight gain. Has your baby been gaining well? If so, you're okay.

If you pump, don't make the mistake of thinking the amount you're producing in a pump session is what baby would have received at breast. Babies are much better than breast pumps at milk removal.

Some moms also worry their supply is low because they notice their baby goes longer stretches between feeds when getting a bottle-feed. There are a few reasons for this. Breastfeeding is more work for your baby than bottle-feeding, and because your breastmilk is on a 24-hour cycle (typically more in the morning), breastfed babies get variable feeds throughout the day.

The bottom line is, breastfeeding and bottle-feeding are apples and oranges. When evaluating your supply, look first at your baby's weight.

## WHY SUPPLY IS LOW

The most common reason for low supply is lack of milk removal. Mom may not be feeding or pumping enough for various reasons, or the baby isn't effectively removing milk from the breasts. Often this happens when mom and baby experienced a difficult birth or postpartum complications, or there is a lack of breast-feeding support and education available to the family.

Many moms worry their supply is decreasing because of their diet or dehydration. As long as you are not malnourished, dehydrated, or losing more than 1.5 pounds a week, a dip in supply is most likely not because of your diet or hydration.

Usually, a low breastmilk supply is the result of insufficient milk removal and stimulation. Other factors include hormonal imbalances, certain medications, anemia, postpartum hemorrhage, retained placenta, prior breast surgeries, formula supplementation, and polycystic ovarian syndrome (PCOS). Discuss any of these conditions with your healthcare provider as soon as possible.

## THREE TIPS TO INCREASE SUPPLY

If you think your supply is low, reach out to an LC (either locally or virtually) as soon as possible. Your LC will take a medical history, and together you'll come up with a plan to increase your supply. Try not to use the advice from a friend or what you're seeing online. Each plan of care is specifically tailored to a particular mom and baby. Most medical insurance plans will cover LCs, and if you're not insured, many offer sliding scales or payment options.

Having said that, here are some general tips for increasing supply:

### Increase Feeding Frequency

Are you removing milk from your breasts a minimum of 8 to 12 times every 24 hours? Try encouraging your baby to cluster feed (feed, say, every 30 or 60 minutes). Babies naturally want to cluster feed in the late afternoon or evening, which can give your supply a quick boost. Also, make sure you're not going too long at night without feeding or pumping. For some moms, dropping the middle-of-the-night feed adversely affects their supply.

### Pump after Feeding

Inserting an extra pump session after breastfeeding is another quick way to give your supply a little boost. To do this, pump both breasts for 10 minutes right after the breastfeed. Some moms like to wait 30 to 45 minutes after the feed, but if you go that route, be careful. Ideally, you don't want to pump right before your next breastfeed. Try to do that "extra" pump session in the morning, because you'll probably be able to pump more milk then. More bang for your buck!

### Eat Lactogenic Foods

When it comes to diet, you want to make sure you're getting enough calories. Listening to your body and eating to hunger and drinking to thirst is fine for most women. There's no need to count calories. If you suspect you're not eating enough, try to sneak in calorie-rich foods like nuts and add sauces to your meals.

Additionally, women have used specific foods to boost their milk supply for centuries, such as apricots, barley, brewer's yeast, dark or leafy greens, dates, fennel seed, legumes, moringa, and oatmeal.

## Supplementing Your Supply

Not all moms are able to establish a full supply. And that's okay. Acknowledge that you're working hard and that breastfeeding can be a really tough road. Any breastmilk you're able to give your baby is beneficial, and you need to make the choice that's best *for you, your family, and your mental health.* Fun fact: Moms typically have more milk with each baby. If you have another baby, you'll probably produce more the second time around.

Supplementing your breastmilk can take many different forms. You might be pumping your own milk, or using donor milk or formula. Let's take a look at each of these options.

### SUPPLEMENTING WITH PUMPED MILK

If you're going to pump and supplement with your own breastmilk, you'll want to use a quality home-grade pump or hospital-grade pump (usually available as rentals). Try pumping when your baby gets a full bottle-feed *and* right after some breastfeeds. The more you pump, the more breastmilk you'll have to supplement with—*and* the extra milk removal and stimulation should boost your supply. Remember, your milk supply is responsive. It's all about demand and supply. Make sure you're also using your hands to massage the breasts and help with expression because that maximizes output and often results in greater production. But be careful—overdoing pumping frequency is definitely possible and may lead to sore nipples.

## SUPPLEMENTING WITH DONOR MILK

Using donor milk means you are still feeding your baby breast-milk, just from another mom. There are a few ways to acquire donor milk. If you decide to go this route, research each option, speak to your pediatrician, evaluate risks and benefits, and decide what a good fit is for you.

Milk banks are one way to get donor milk. They collect breast-milk, pasteurize it, and sell it to hospitals and families. Breastmilk donors are typically screened, and the pasteurization process eliminates anything that might be harmful in the milk.

Peer-to-peer milk donation is a more informal way of getting breastmilk and is often coordinated online. With this type of milk donation, requests for health history and drop-off or pick up arrangements are typically made between two families once they connect. Another option is breastmilk donations from family or friends who are breastfeeding.

Donations (either peer-to-peer or from family or friends) raise the risk of milk contamination, which could make your child sick. If you choose this option, explore the risks and be sure to discuss your plans with your pediatrician.

## SUPPLEMENTING WITH FORMULA

Supplementing breastfeeding with formula is called combo-feeding. Some families choose this route because mom has difficulty establishing a full supply, it's medically necessary, or this is just what works best.

A couple of things to keep in mind when combo-feeding: Formula tends to be a little more constipating. You'll notice your baby's stools are more formed and smellier (sorry!). Also, formula will sometimes keep your baby full longer because it takes longer for the baby's body to digest. While studies show that breast-feeding parents sleep longer at night, some may find that giving a formula bottle as the last feed of the night helps their baby sleep longer. Of course, sleeping for longer stretches at night sometimes reduces milk supply, so watch your baby and your breasts to see how they do when you try a new plan.

## PACED BOTTLE-FEEDING

If you're supplementing beyond the first week or two, going back to work, or just want an occasional date night, chances are you're going to be using a bottle. If so, it's very important to use the "paced bottle-feeding" technique, a method also recommended by the American Academy of Pediatrics for bottle-feeding any baby.

Follow these tips to give a bottle using paced bottle-feeding:

Use a slow-flow nipple.

Use an age-appropriate amount of breastmilk (from three weeks on, that's three to four ounces).

Place baby in a sitting position or reclined up to 45 degrees.

Run the bottle over baby's nose and lips and wait for an open mouth.

Insert the nipple into the baby's mouth at the back of the hard palate (i.e., all the way in their mouth) once baby opens.

Hold the bottle as horizontal to the floor as possible, keeping nipple full as baby sucks.

Allow the baby to feed for 15 to 30 seconds, then tilt the bottle up in their mouth. Alternatively, remove the bottle from their mouth at this time and let the nipple touch their lips.

Watch for baby to catch their breath AND cue they are ready for more. They will probably open wide or shake their head.

Return to feeding for 15 to 30 seconds and repeat.

A full bottle-feed should take about 10 to 15 minutes and feel "controlled," with no choking, gagging, or milk leaking out of the side of baby's mouth.

Toward the end of the feed, when you take a break, you may notice baby catch their breath but not cue that they want more. That's your baby saying they are done. Don't nudge them to finish the bottle.

Using paced bottle-feeding is important for several reasons:

It mimics the way the breast releases milk, so it helps prevent bottle "preferencing" (a.k.a. "nipple confusion").

It's much more natural for the baby because we naturally drink in "waves."

It prevents lots of gulping, which cuts down on gas.

It's responsive. We know that some of the health benefits of breastfeeding for baby (lower rates of obesity, heart disease, and diabetes) are partially due to a baby self-regulating their intake. We don't want to undo those benefits by nudging a baby to finish a bottle.

Remember that supplementing is all about finding the method that works best for you and your family. If something isn't working (or stops working), don't be afraid to switch it up.

# 21 Troubleshooting Tips

**U**h oh! Did something go wrong? Take a breath. You *will* encounter issues while on your breastfeeding journey, and that's super normal! Almost all speed bumps are temporary issues that can be resolved quickly. Some require a more official game plan. Either way, we've got this, mama! You have lots of resources (including this book) available to you. The key is understanding what's going on and getting professional help when necessary. Ask your pediatrician. Reach out to your LC. Find a local breastfeeding support group. Search out your local La Leche League meeting. All are good resources to get you back on the right track.

# Tips

This section focuses on troubleshooting some of the most common breastfeeding and other related issues. As you progress through the weeks and months ahead, revisit this chapter any time you hit a new obstacle or challenge that's stressing you out.

## ALLERGIC REACTIONS

Babies can have allergic reactions to the proteins from food in your diet, but it's not as common as most people think. Don't start by radically changing your diet. Food elimination diets are difficult and inconvenient, so don't begin one casually. Most of the time, if your baby has excessive gas or discomfort in the first few weeks, it's a growth spurt and not what you're eating. When there's an allergy, your pediatrician will typically review the symptoms and take a stool sample to test for traces of blood. Don't avoid any foods unless your pediatrician or LC has created that plan for you.

## BABY CHOKES WHILE EATING (OVERSUPPLY)

Fast flow means lots of milk. Sometimes babies have difficulty controlling the flow, especially if it's around peak milk time (usually in the morning). Try moving your baby from a horizontal feeding position (see "Cradle Hold" on page 26) to a diagonal feeding position (see "Laid-Back Hold" on page 29) where the head is higher than the feet. This is called a "gravitational position" and gives the baby more control over the flow. You might also try hand expressing (or using a hand pump) to express a little milk off the first let-down. If these tips don't work, you may need to work with an LC to reduce your supply a little.

## BABY CRIES AND ARCHES BACK AFTER FEEDING

If your baby is under six weeks old and arching their back, it may be gas from a growth spurt. But if your baby is older than six weeks, appears to be in pain at the end of a feed, is inconsolable, frequently spits up, arches their back, has poor weight gain, and doesn't like being laid down flat, you should ask your pediatrician about GERD (gastroesophageal reflux disease). It's also helpful to record a video of your baby crying after a feed, so you can show your pediatrician what you're experiencing at home.

## BABY REJECTS BOTTLE

Babies typically reject the bottle for a few reasons. First, they aren't receiving it frequently enough. For many babies, the bottle needs to be part of their daily routine or they will decide they don't want it anymore. Another culprit is teething. If a baby's gums hurt, they may reject the bottle. Try offering relief measures, like rubbing their gums or using a teething ring, before offering the bottle (see "Teething and Biting" on page 134). Another reason could be an issue with the milk. Does it smell funny or bad? (See "Baby Rejects Frozen Milk" below.)

The key to a "bottle strike" is to identify the underlying cause (if you can) and keep offering the bottle on a regular basis.

## BABY REJECTS FROZEN MILK

Some moms have excess lipase (an enzyme) in their breastmilk that causes changes to their milk once frozen. Before you freeze lots of breastmilk, make sure you defrost a bag and check it out. Smell it to make sure it doesn't have an odd or weird (soapy or metallic) scent. If you do detect this odor, try the fairly easy fix called flash-scalding where you heat the milk to 80 to 90°F (but don't boil it) before freezing.

If you have frozen milk with excess lipase, try giving it to your baby anyway. It's not a problem if your baby doesn't care. If your baby rejects the milk because they don't like the taste, you can also try combining the frozen with some freshly expressed breastmilk.

## BABY WON'T SLEEP

This is such a tough one, and solutions really depend on how old your baby is. If baby is under six weeks, it's expected they won't sleep for long stretches. Young babies are nocturnal, and frequent growth spurts may keep you up with all-night marathon feedings. If baby is between two to four months, what are you defining as "won't sleep"? Nighttime sleep at this age most commonly looks like a four- to six-hour stretch, a feed, then a two- to three-hour stretch. If baby is older than 16 weeks and weighs more than 16 pounds, it may be time to do some research and put together a sleep plan that fits your parenting style. As you try out different techniques, stick with each one for a while before giving up on it. The key is consistency.

## BACK AND SHOULDER PAIN

Are you leaning over to feed your baby? Bringing your breast to your baby? Or looking down at that adorable face throughout the feed?

Make sure you always bring baby to you. If you're using a breastfeeding pillow, place it right under your breast. You'll most likely also need a bed pillow between the breastfeeding pillow and your lap.

Take regular breaks to roll your neck and shoulders and try not to stare at (your gorgeous) baby the whole time you are feeding.

You might also consider completely switching up the breastfeeding position you're using. Have you tried leaning back while breastfeeding (see "Laid-Back Hold" on page 29) or turning on your side (see "Side-Lying Hold" on page 30)?

## BOTTLE-FEEDING DOS AND DON'TS

- Do use paced bottle-feeding (see "Paced Bottle-Feeding" on page 40).
- Do make sure everyone who bottle-feeds baby uses the same technique.
- Do use a slow-flow nipple.
- Do hold baby at a 45-degree angle.
- Do use an appropriate amount of milk.
- Do experiment with bottles to see which one works best for baby.
- Do watch baby's cues to see when they are done feeding.
- Don't let baby drink too fast.
- Don't give up if baby doesn't like the bottle at first.
- Don't prop the bottle.
- Don't ignore baby while bottle-feeding.
- Don't nudge baby to finish a bottle once they are done.

## BREASTFEEDING WHILE SICK

If you're sick, stay hydrated and continue to feed your baby. There are very few situations where it's not best to keep breastfeeding. Continuing to breastfeed your baby provides them with specific antibodies that helps boost their immune system and protect them from germs in their environment. Check with your physician or LC if you're not sure.

If baby is sick, you may notice more frequent, shorter feeds, especially if their nose is stuffy or it's hard for them to breathe. They may also be doing more "comfort sucking" because they don't feel good. Monitor baby's daily wet diaper count and stay in touch with your pediatrician.

## CESAREAN RECOVERY

A cesarean birth is major surgery.

You may be separated from baby right after birth. You may or may not be able to have that early "golden hour" breastfeed. Don't worry—just breastfeed as soon as you're together. If you're going to be separated from baby for 12 hours or more, ask for a hospital-grade pump so you can start pumping.

You may be tender around your incision. When feeding, use positions that move baby off your torso (see "Football or Clutch Hold" on page 28). Your doctor will most likely prescribe pain medication. If they know you're breastfeeding, they'll give you medications compatible with breastfeeding. Controlling your pain is important. Many moms report that when they're feeling discomfort from the cesarean surgery, breastfeeding is more uncomfortable too.

With cesarean births, a mom's milk may transition from colostrum to transitional milk a little later. You're a little more likely, then, to need to give formula for a short period of time, perhaps a day or two, until your milk transitions. This is usually on a short-term basis, though.

Once home, you will probably need some assistance moving around, getting baby set up for breastfeeding, and taking care of yourself. Line up a support system, ask for help, and try not to push yourself too hard.

### CLOGGED DUCT SIGNS AND TREATMENT

A clogged or plugged duct usually feels like a hard, tender area inside your breast and causes sharp, shooting pains that increase in intensity over time. It happens when milk coagulates and gets stuck in the ductal network. To clear a plug, you need to break it up. Try Epsom salt soaks followed by suction, breast massage, and dangle feeding (where you lean over baby and let gravity help out).

Plugged ducts can happen for many reasons, including going a longer stretch of time without feeding or pumping, wearing an underwire bra, carrying a heavy bag or backpack, compressing the same area of your breast for a period of time, or having oversupply. Sometimes you'll never know what caused the clog. It might be the internal anatomy of your breast or something you have no control over.

When you have a plug, be sure to aggressively work to clear it. If the clog doesn't resolve within a couple of days, it can turn into mastitis.

### COMBO-FEEDING (BREASTMILK AND FORMULA)

Combo-feeding is giving your baby breastmilk and formula. Some families choose this plan intentionally because it works for them, and others combo-feed because mom hasn't been able to establish a full supply, baby is not gaining weight at a rate the pediatrician is happy with, or for other medical reasons.

Finding a formula that works for your baby can sometimes take experimentation. Formulas can be dairy-based, soy-based, organic, or made of "predigested" or hydrolyzed protein. In addition to base ingredients, formulas also come in a variety of forms, such as ready-to-feed, concentrated, and powdered. Talk to your pediatrician about the best choice for your baby.

If you are introducing formula into your baby's diet for the first time, you may notice that the stooling frequency slows down, and that the stool is more formed and smellier. This is very normal.

## ENGORGEMENT (SWOLLEN BREASTS)

When your milk transitions between days three and five, you may experience uncomfortable fullness in your breasts. This is called "initial engorgement" and typically lasts one to two days. Some moms don't experience any engorgement, and that is also normal.

If you are engorged, cold compresses are your primary remedy. Apply bags of frozen peas or corn to your breast tissue—on for 15 minutes, off for 15 minutes, and back on for 15 minutes—throughout the day. Continue breastfeeding your baby. And if you still find that you're uncomfortably full, you can pump *just enough* to take the edge off. Don't do a full pump session, as that tells your body to send more milk and will make the engorgement worse.

## FEELING EXHAUSTED ALL THE TIME

Taking care of a baby is exhausting. Make sure you're taking care of you too. Are you eating? Getting outside? Eating regular meals? If not, call in your support network to give you some relief so you can look after yourself.

Keep an eye on your mental health. Perinatal (the period surrounding birth) depression is one of the most common complications of pregnancy (and not talked about nearly enough). It can show up as exhaustion, sadness that doesn't pass, or thoughts of hurting yourself or baby. If you suspect you might have postpartum depression or anxiety, you can call Postpartum Support International at 1-800-944-4773 for help in English or Spanish or go to Postpartum.net.

## FEELING ISOLATED

Having a newborn can be an isolating experience, especially if you are a single parent or have a partner who returned to work.

Find a local breastfeeding support group or new parent meet-up and commit to getting out of the house. Most likely you'll meet people and end up forming a circle of friends. If attending a class or group feels like too much, try putting the baby in the stroller and walking to the park or the mall. You may find other new parents doing the same thing.

If you can't get out of the house, try connecting with other parents online (see "Mom Groups Online" on page 9). Social media groups can be a great source of support and friendship.

## GROWTH SPURTS

Babies typically have four growth spurts in the first six weeks. They arrive around days 2 or 3 (usually starts the second night and lasts a couple of days), days 7 to 10 (lasts a couple of days), days 14 to 21 (lasts about a week), and between 4 to 6 weeks (lasts about a week). The three-week and six-week growth spurts are usually pretty intense. After those, you'll probably see growth spurts again for a week around the top of three months, four months, six months, nine months, and twelve months.

What does a growth spurt look like?

+ Cranky baby who is very hard to soothe

+ Baby feeds more frequently and more voraciously

+ Baby cues to feed *all the time*, even right after a feed

+ Baby's sleep pattern changes. Baby may be waking up all night, every hour. (Or nights are okay, but daytime is a feeding frenzy.)

+ Very gassy baby

+ Baby may have preference for the bottle

+ Baby has TONS of wet diapers

+ Baby may spit up more

+ Mom's nipples may be more sore

+ If mom finds time to pump, her volumes may be down because baby is feeding so frequently

+ Parents are exhausted

Here's what to do:

+ Feed the baby a minimum of 8 to 12 times every 24 hours, but try not to overfeed. (Lots of spit-up can be a sign that baby is overfeeding.)

+ Provide gas relief. Try using regular doses of infant gas drops (with simethicone) and tummy massage (see "Constipation" on page 116).

+ Wear the baby. Putting the baby in a wrap can be a lifesaver, especially during growth spurts.

+ Give the pacifier (if introduced) or a finger (pad side–up) for baby to suck on, especially after a feed.

+ Remind yourself this is normal and will pass.

If you are worried about your baby, see your pediatrician for a weight check. Babies often gain a lot (one ounce per day or more) during growth spurts.

When bottle-feeding, remember that a baby will often take whatever you offer. How much they take in a bottle is NOT an indicator of how much they needed or how hungry they were. Use paced bottle-feeding (see "Paced Bottle-Feeding" on page 40).

You will know your baby is done with the growth spurt when they appear more relaxed, demand fewer feeds, and life gets easier.

## LATCHING HURTS

Latching may be uncomfortable for the first couple of weeks as you and baby master this new skill. But it should not make you cry or dread breastfeeding. If latching hurts, go back to the basics—use the cross-cradle hold and work on your deep-latch technique (see "Cross-Cradle Hold" on page 27 and "How to Get a Good Latch" on page 20).

If you've tried different techniques and your nipples are still hurting, reach out to your LC or find a local breastfeeding support group.

If you've got the basics down, and your nipples are still very damaged or sore, your baby may have a tongue-tie, which makes breastfeeding properly difficult (see "Tongue-Tied" on page 24).

## MILK HASN'T TRANSITIONED YET

Your milk should transition from colostrum to transitional milk around days three to five. If this transition doesn't happen, ask your obstetrician if you may have retained placenta. Your doctor may do an ultrasound to check. Having a portion of your placenta still in your uterus will keep your milk from transitioning.

Losing a lot of blood during birth (Sheehan's syndrome) can also cause your milk to transition later.

If both have been ruled out, and it's been more than five days, insert a few extra daily pump sessions (in addition to breastfeeding) and reach out to your LC or local breastfeeding support group.

## PACIFIER DOS AND DON'TS

+ Do try to wait until breastfeeding is established to offer a pacifier.

+ Do start with a pacifier that has a long, narrow nipple. This shape replicates nipple position in a baby's mouth during breastfeeding.

+ Do keep nipples up-to-date by age recommendation. An older baby could bite off the tip of a pacifier, which is a choking hazard.

+ Don't let the pacifier cover hunger cues. If you introduce a pacifier and the baby has less than eight feeds a day, stop using it.

+ Don't use a pacifier if the baby is having weight gain issues.

+ Don't introduce a pacifier unless you feel it is really needed. Studies show that babies who take a pacifier wean sooner and get more middle ear infections than babies who don't.

## PUMPING HURTS

Pumping should not hurt! It might feel a bit weird the first few times, but it shouldn't hurt or leave you with sore nipples.

Make sure you're not turning the vacuum or suction up too high. You should always use the highest comfortable setting. *If it hurts, turn it down.* More is not better.

Also, are you using the correct size flange? Flanges come in many sizes. The flange should draw in your nipple and a little bit of your areola. Look at what's happening at the end of the pumping session. If your nipple is rubbing up against the sides of the "tunnel," the flange is too small.

Finally, are you using a good pump? There are good pumps, and there are bad pumps that can cause nipple damage. Look for a double electric pump that gets lots of great reviews from other pumping moms who are breastfeeding. Ask friends, ask online, and look at posted reviews. If you're not sure which pump is best for you, reach out to an LC or breastfeeding support group for pump advice.

## THRUSH

Are you experiencing very itchy breasts, with pink, flaky, shiny skin? Does baby have a thick white coating on their tongue or inside their cheeks and a diaper rash? If so, the source of discomfort might be thrush, a fungal infection that requires a prescription for you and baby. You'll also need to sterilize bottles, pacifiers, and pump parts daily.

Thrush can be difficult to resolve, and sometimes requires changes in your diet or alternative treatments. Speak to your obstetrician or pediatrician if you suspect either of you has thrush.

## Summary

These are some of the most common breastfeeding issues, but this list is in no way comprehensive. Many things could be happening with you and your baby. Above all, trust your instincts, and if you feel like there might be a serious problem, seek out your pediatrician or lactation consultant. Take note of any of the strategies you've tried so you can provide as much information as possible when discussing your baby. It always helps medical providers when they know more about your situation. And remember there is no right way to breastfeed except the one that works for you and your family.

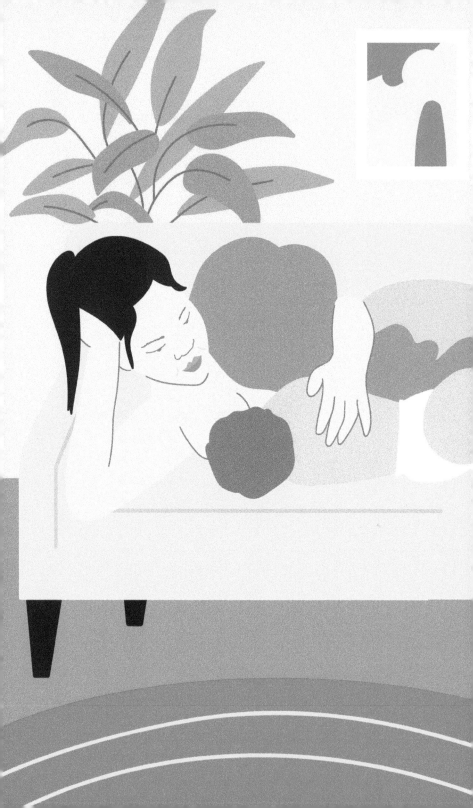

# PART TWO

# Months 1 to 6

## First Month

Congratulations! Your baby has arrived and now it's go time. You've spent months wondering what life will be like with your baby, and now that your little one is here, they are *ready to feed* (and feed, and feed). For most parents, this first month feels like a blur of emotions, diapers, feeds, and hours that melt together as you learn about each other. Here's the inside scoop: The first six weeks are usually the hardest, and it generally gets easier after that. But we're going to break it down, take it step by step, and get through this together.

So why are the first few weeks usually the hardest? Bottom line, there's *a lot* happening. You're probably recovering from birth, you and your baby are both learning how to feed, baby is having multiple growth spurts (see "Growth Spurts" on page 50), your schedule is tied to your baby's nocturnal sleep cycle, and the sleep deprivation is hard-core. In the best of circumstances, this time can be very challenging. Here's the good news: Your body has been preparing for this day and your baby has inborn instincts that will help you both through the first month.

## Monthly Goal #1:
## Learn to Latch: Practice. Practice. Practice.

For most moms and babies, practice is the name of the game. While you're busy focusing on techniques to get a deep, pain-free latch (see "How to Get a Good Latch" on page 20), your baby is learning how to feed and coordinate the suck, swallow, breathe rhythm, which is tricky stuff. A good latch may take time to figure out. How long could be anywhere from a few days to a few weeks. Sidenote: If you're a mom who finds that latching is a breeze from the beginning, that's awesome!

## Monthly Goal #2: Find Your Favorite Position

The breastfeeding positions you're using in the hospital during the first few days may be very different than the ones you'll eventually use at home. As you find the positions that work well for you (see "Assume the Position" on page 25) this month, try to keep these general principles in mind. Always bring baby to you instead of leaning over and bringing your breast to the baby.

And remember to take some breaks from staring at your baby's beautiful face by stretching your neck and rolling your shoulders. These two good habits will help protect your back and neck. Finally, there's no absolute right and wrong when it comes to breastfeeding positions. A good breastfeeding position prevents aches and pains, helps protect against sore nipples, and gets baby to relax into the feed and transfer milk.

## Monthly Goal #3: Establish a Strong Supply

Your body is *actively* trying to figure out how much milk to make. How frequently (and effectively) you remove milk from your breast is the *main factor* that determines how much milk you make. Your body is expecting a minimum of 8 to 12 feeds every 24 hours to establish a full milk supply. (If you're having trouble keeping your supply up, see "Three Tips to Increase Supply" on page 36.)

## Monthly Goal #4:
## Surround Yourself with Support

A big challenge for you this month is that babies are often nocturnal for the first few weeks, *and* they are moving in and out of growth spurts (which make for intense feeding days) that can be hard on everyone. Support can make the difference between feeling like you're barely surviving to actually catching your breath every once in a while. Help takes many forms. Sometimes the challenge is figuring out exactly what kind of support you need, *and* deciding what isn't helping you.

# Week #1

**Weekly Goal #1: Latch**—*Aim to get the first breastfeed in right after birth.* We call this time "the golden hour," and we know that when baby does this early feed, breastfeeding tends to go better for both mom and baby. The nurse or midwife who is present during the birth will help you. If you had a cesarean or complication during birth, it may be a few hours until you and baby are able to feed. Don't worry; just do your first breastfeed as soon as you're back together.

**Weekly Goal #2: Positions**—*Try the football hold.* In the hospital, this position (see "Football or Clutch Hold" on page 28) often works well because it helps both you and your support staff see baby's latch and make adjustments. It also gets baby off your torso, which may be tender in the days following birth.

**Weekly Goal #3: Supply**—If your baby is being supplemented with a bottle, *start pumping.* If you don't have a good double-electric pump (see "The Big Breastfeeding Checklist" on page 12), hand expression is a great alternative. Aim to do one full pump session for each full bottle your baby is given.

**Weekly Goal #4: Support**—*Find a local Lactation Consultant who comes highly recommended.* The job of LCs is to support you, and they are often covered by your medical insurance. LCs don't just help with latching and positioning. They also provide education on pumping, bottle-feeding, healing, milk supply, and what's normal at each stage. They also support families who choose combo-feeding (breastmilk and formula) as well as those who are exclusively pumping.

**Milestone: The Demand**—You need to feed your baby when your baby shows signs of hunger. You'll also need to make sure you're feeding your baby a minimum of 8 to 12 times each day. It's very common for newborns to feed on the more frequent end of that range. Before your milk transitions, you'll probably feed the baby every 2 ½ to 3 hours, start to start, around the clock. For the first few days, a full feed is 10 to 15 minutes on each breast.

---

**KEY ADVICE: GET TO KNOW YOUR BABY**

*Did you know your baby is hardwired to communicate with you? You'll start to notice your baby showing you feeding cues like putting their hands in their mouth, rooting, and bobbing up and down on your chest (see "How You'll Know Baby Is Hungry" on page 18). Offering a breastfeed when you get those early cues is called "feeding on demand." Meanwhile, your team of doctors, midwives, and nurses will be monitoring your baby's output. This is an awesome time to download an app to track feeds, wet diapers, and stools.*

---

**Milestone: The Gains**—Babies typically lose weight in the first few days. If your baby loses 10 percent or more of their birth weight, your pediatrician will most likely ask you to supplement. You can do this with formula or your own breastmilk. Either way, if you're supplementing, you'll need to start pumping to protect your supply and encourage your milk to transition (see "Biology Basics" on page 2).

## BREASTFEEDING A PREMATURE BABY

Sometimes babies arrive earlier than planned. If this happens to you, take comfort in knowing you will be *surrounded* by a team of providers who will care for you and for your baby. Ask your NICU team when it might be possible for you to do kangaroo care with your baby (holding your baby skin to skin). This contact stabilizes baby's temperature and breathing, and helps conserve calories. Most premature babies will need time to learn how to breastfeed, and in the meantime, you'll need to pump your breastmilk to establish and protect your supply. Ideally, you should start pumping within six hours of baby's birth. We typically recommend a hospital-grade pump for the first month or two. You'll be pumping both breasts approximately every three hours for 15 minutes.

Also very important is that everyone feeding your baby uses the paced bottle-feeding technique, so your baby doesn't become "preferenced" to a fast bottle flow. Ask the NICU nurses or LC to show you paced bottle-feeding (see "Paced Bottle-Feeding" on page 40).

Check with your NICU team for their policies on providing pumped breastmilk to your baby as well as storage and transport requirements. When your baby is ready to start breastfeeding, you may find a nipple shield or a supplementary nursing system (SNS)—a feeding tube device to help with supplemental feeds at the breast—helpful to support your baby as they learn this new skill. Be sure to request a visit from an LC. They will help you latch the baby, suggest needed tools, and help establish the best plan to help you meet your goal. Your baby is going to need time to ramp up and learn the skills needed to become good at breastfeeding. As long as you establish and protect your supply, and have a plan in place to support baby, your goals should still be within reach.

## Week #2

**Weekly Goal #1: Latch—***Focus on having baby open their mouth (WIDE) before latching on.* Start by expressing a drop of breast-milk on your nipple, then running your nipple over the baby's nose and lips. Get that BIG, OPEN WIDE mouth before latching. The more open your baby's mouth is before latching, the more likely you are to get a deep, comfortable latch.

---

**KEY ADVICE: FUN FACT**

*By this week, your breastmilk has transitioned from colostrum to transitional milk. Your milk supply will continue to increase over the next few weeks.*

---

**Weekly Goal #2: Positions—***Focus on using the cross-cradle and football holds (see "Cross-Cradle Hold" and "Football or Clutch Hold" on pages 27 and 28).* In these positions, you're placing a strong hand behind baby's ears, neck, and back, and you'll hold them firmly in place so they don't lose that deep latch.

**Milestone: The Demand**—Once the milk transitions, moms with an average to strong supply should offer one breast. Do a nice, full feed, then top off with the second breast, if needed. Sometimes baby will take one breast at a feed, and sometimes they'll take two. Around day seven, you may notice that baby wants to feed *a lot*. They may also be extra gassy and cranky. Hello, growth spurt. This should last a couple of days.

**Weekly Goal #3: Supply**—Milk removal is an important factor in establishing your supply. *Experiment with using the side of your hand or your thumb to do breast massage while you breast-feed.* Move the milk from the top of your breast to about halfway down. You'll see baby feed more actively. Another method is to use your hand to compress a full area of your breast while feeding. Both of these techniques will nudge a sleepy baby to feed better, make the breastfeed more efficient, and facilitate milk removal, which leads to a stronger supply.

**Weekly Goal #4: Support**—Friends and family will most likely ask how they can help. *Start that running "help me" list of what you need, so you can hand out tasks when people ask.* Maybe it's a meal train, a supportive phone call, a run to the store, a quick visit to hold baby so you can nap or shower, or even a household chore like washing the dishes.

**Milestone: The Gains**—Now that your milk has transitioned, your baby should be gaining approximately 5.5 to 8 ounces per week. If your pediatrician isn't happy with your baby's weight gain, they may recommend that you reach out to an LC to work on your supply and feeding issues. The goal is for baby to return to their birth weight by day 14, although sometimes this gain can take a little longer.

## Week #3

**Weekly Goal #1: Latch**—Don't stay in a bad latch. *If the latch hurts, break the latch and try again.* To break the latch, insert your index finger or pinky into baby's mouth, between their gums, and scoop your nipple out. If you just pull baby off the breast without breaking the latch first, it can damage your nipple.

**Weekly Goal #2: Positions**—*Experiment with positions.* Besides discovering a new position that may work better for you and baby, switching positions helps your nipples be more comfortable. Have you tried laid-back breastfeeding yet? (See "Laid-Back Hold" on page 29.)

**Weekly Goal #3: Supply**—*Follow your baby's lead.* This week your baby will probably want to do lots of snacking. You may find you're doing about 12 feeds a day instead of 8 to 10, and that's super normal during a growth spurt. All this frequent feeding is going to give your supply a natural boost this week.

**Milestone: The Demand**— During the three-week growth spurt (it arrives around days 14 to 21), your baby is not only going to want to feed often, but you may also notice their sleep pattern is off (most likely lots of night feeds) and they are getting TONS of wet diapers. Hang in there; this one will last about a week.

**Weekly Goal #4: Support**—Many families will tell you this week is one of the hardest, making it a great time to call in support, wherever it's available. *If you live with a partner, talk about how you can tag-team to give each other a break.* Maybe you take turns taking daytime naps, so you're both ready for the marathon nights. If that's not possible, there are lots of ways for your partner to help with the breastfeeding (see "Your Partner" on page 8). Most of all, HANG IN THERE!

**Milestone: The Gains**—Your baby may gain close to one ounce a day this week. That's the three-week growth spurt in action.

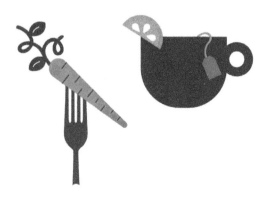

*A breastfeeding mom's body needs approximately 300 to 500 additional calories per day to support the production of a full supply. Try to eat three meals plus snacks throughout the day. Create a few "stations" in the places where you breastfeed frequently, and stock them with water and snacks that are easy to eat with one hand. There are no specific foods you need to eat or drink while breastfeeding. Drink to thirst and eat frequently. This isn't a good time to restrict your calories or to actively diet.*

## Week #4

**Weekly Goal #1: Latch**—Is baby choking or gagging on your milk flow in the morning? Many moms notice their supply is stronger in the morning and may be a little fast for baby. If so, *try hand expressing a little milk before latching to take the edge off that morning let-down.* (Tip: A hand pump works great here too.)

**Weekly Goal #2: Positions**—Is baby able to maintain a deep latch on their own now? *Try moving to cradle position* (see "Cradle Hold" on page 26). Doesn't that feel better? Now you have a free hand for your phone, the remote control, or a snack.

**Milestone: The Gains**—Baby should still be steadily gaining 5.5 to 8 ounces per week. Weight gain is one of the most important tools your medical team uses to determine how your baby is doing.

**Weekly Goal #3: Supply**—Did you know that women have been eating oats to increase milk supply for centuries? If you're an oatmeal fan, *try eating steel-cut oats (not instant) once a day and see if you notice a difference.* Overnight oats are an easy way to make them. Prepare them ahead of time, and toss in some fruit or chocolate chips for a little extra fun. If this seems like a big feat right now, ask your partner to make oats or add it to your running "help me" list.

---

**KEY ADVICE: HEALTH AND WELLNESS**

*You may be feeling some shifts in your mood over the next few weeks. It's very normal to experience baby blues, which can be triggered by fluctuating hormones, sleep deprivation, stress—all the changes that can accompany becoming a new parent. You may experience intense mood swings, crying, irritability, and inability to sleep. Have you been getting out of the house? A walk around the block (with baby in the stroller) or by yourself can do wonders for your mental health.*

---

**Weekly Goal #4: Support**—Postpartum doulas are awesome resources. They will come to your home and assist with everything from newborn care basics, light household chores, night feeds, and parent education. *Ask your friends and families for referrals, search online, or post on social media for recommendations.*

**Milestone: The Demands**—You're probably *so relieved* to be done with the week three growth spurt. This week should feel a lot calmer, and a return to the pattern that existed before last week. Your baby is now eating approximately 8 times a day, instead of 12 (or more). High fives all around—you survived!

*Baby's average daily breastmilk intake has plateaued by now. It's super counterintuitive (you were thinking bigger, older baby needs more milk, right?), but the average daily intake plateaus around 3 weeks at 19 to 32 ounces per day, with the average around 25 ounces per day. That's great news for you and should take a ton of pressure off. You won't need to make more and more (and more) milk as baby gets older. Breastmilk changes in composition, caloric content, and fat content as baby's rate of growth changes, but the amount they take every day will remain constant until it slowly starts decreasing with the addition of solids around six months.*

# Second Month

You made it to month two! This month should feel *much* calmer. You and baby are probably starting to get into a nice groove with breastfeeding, and it might all be starting to feel a little bit easier. Some people call this month the "reward period." Thank goodness, right?

At this point, breastfeeding is considered established. You and baby should have a good handle on latching, so we can go ahead and integrate new skills and techniques that will give you and your family more flexibility.

## Monthly Goal #1: Express Yourself! Learn to Pump

For most families, four to six weeks is the perfect time to introduce pumping and bottle-feeding. (If you introduced it earlier, don't worry; you just got a jump start on this step. You can use this month to fine-tune your pumping and bottle-feeding skills.) For most moms, a new high-quality home-grade pump is essential (see "The Big Breastfeeding Checklist" on page 12), but some moms find hand expression even easier and more effective. Honestly, hand expression is a great skill to have in your toolbox if you're outside the house without your pump, or you just need to quickly express a little milk and move on.

## Monthly Goal #2: Introduce a Bottle

Once you've started pumping, you can introduce breastmilk in a bottle. Of course, you can also bottle-feed with formula, and that's *absolutely* the right choice for many families. Either way, you're going to want to use the paced bottle-feeding method (see "Paced Bottle-Feeding" on page 40). With this technique, you'll use a slow-flow nipple, hold baby in a semi-reclined (45-degree angle) position, give the milk slowly in controlled "waves," and be responsive to your baby's body language.

## Monthly Goal #3: Find Your Village

It's time to get out there and find your people. For centuries, we lived together in villages supporting one another and passing down valuable knowledge from generation to generation. You might be feeling a very real need to connect with others around this time. That's super normal. All support people in your life are essential, but having another mom who has been there or is currently going through the same things you are is *invaluable*. You may make friends who help you through this season in your life, and in the process of supporting one another, you may create very special friendships that last for many years to come. We'll talk about how to find your village.

## Week #1

**Weekly Goal #1: Pumping**—Your new pump will come unassembled, with the parts in bags. First step? *Open the box, take everything out, and sterilize your pump parts.* (Place them in boiling water for about 10 minutes.) Now you're ready to assemble. Some pumps come with easy instructions, and some not so much. You can find helpful videos online, as well as on the pump manufacturer's website. Sometimes partners like to be the ones to own this step and they become the pump expert.

**Weekly Goal #2: Bottle-Feeding**—*Watch a video on paced bottle-feeding this week.* There are a few different techniques, but the main idea is to use a method that is controlled and replicates how the breast works by delivering milk in waves instead of a continuous flow. A full bottle should take about 10 to 15 minutes to feed. If you don't use a paced bottle-feeding technique, babies often discover that the bottle is faster and easier, and they start to prefer it. (They are so smart!)

# NIPPLE CONFUSION

Nipple confusion is a common culprit when a baby has difficulty breastfeeding in the early weeks. Babies get used to the faster flow of the bottle and the feel of the silicone. This is called "preferencing." If possible, avoid giving bottles until breastfeeding is established around four to six weeks. Of course, sometimes babies need bottles in the early days. If your baby needs to be supplemented, make sure you use paced bottle-feeding (see "Paced Bottle-Feeding" on page 40), so baby will continue to go back and forth between bottle and breast.

Pacifiers can be problematic for some babies too. If you introduce a pacifier in the early weeks, watch to make sure it's not covering your baby's hunger cues. If you see the number of feeds in 24 hours decrease, you should remove it. Some moms also observe that the pacifier changes the baby's latch. If you notice that, take it away until your baby is a little older.

**Weekly Goal #3**: Village—Now that baby is a month old, this is the time to get out and *find a local breastfeeding support group or a few of them*. Some groups are moms only, and other groups welcome partners. Some will have a professional scale available, so you can check baby's weight each week and measure how much they take at the breast, whereas others focus on group discussion and education. Almost all support groups will encourage questions and peer support. And most will have a Breastfeeding Educator or LC available to offer advice and professional support. Fees typically range from low cost to free. They are often offered at your local hospital, Lactation Consultant offices, breastfeeding supply stores, and La Leche League. Tip: Don't worry about timing the breastfeed or even feeding while you're at the group.

Many moms come with a full baby or bottle-feed. Just go and see how you like it. Attend a few different ones. You'll know when you've found the one that works for you.

---

**KEY ADVICE: MYTH BUSTED**

*Have you heard that you shouldn't eat spicy foods or foods that cause gas while you're breastfeeding? Well, good news—only in very rare cases are foods truly off limits while you are breastfeeding. Spicy foods and foods that cause you gas cannot cause gas in your baby.*

---

## Week #2

**Weekly Goal #1: Pumping**—Now that your pump is ready to go, and you know how to use it, *let's try pumping for the first time.* There are two common times to pump: either right after a breastfeed or in place of a breastfeed. If you're pumping after a breastfeed, pump both breasts for 10 minutes. If you're pumping in place of a breastfeed, pump both breasts for 15 minutes.

**Weekly Goal #2: Bottle-Feeding**—*And now it's time to offer a bottle.* Once you introduce the bottle, it's a good idea to offer one a day so it's part of the routine, and so your baby will keep taking it. You can offer a full bottle in place of a breastfeed, a "snack" between breastfeeds, or a bottle to break up late afternoon or evening cluster feeding (see "Cluster Feeding" on page 85). Tip: Some babies will take a bottle from mom right from the start, but others won't. A partner, friend, or family member may be the one who has to give the bottle. (By the way, if your baby is particular about who gives the bottle, know that they usually learn to take a bottle from anyone.) If you have a partner at home with you, partners often look forward to this stage because it's a new way for them to bond with baby.

Milestone: Demand—When we talk about breastfeeding babies a minimum of 8 to 12 times every 24 hours, typically 8 times is the most common. But if your baby is in a growth spurt, you may see that number jump up to 10 to 12 times.

Weekly Goal #3: Village—Guess what? You don't actually need to leave your house to find a breastfeeding support group. *Go online and search for virtual support groups.* There are groups on various social media platforms (Facebook, Instagram, etc.) that are likely specific to your location (state, city, or neighborhood) as well as niche groups such as those for exclusive pumping or combo-feeding. A nice advantage to online support groups is that someone is always around at 2 a.m. when you're up for a middle-of-the-night feed.

## Week #3

Weekly Goal #1: Pumping—*Maximize your pump session efficiency this week by experimenting with hands-on pumping.* Dr. Jane Morton researched the effect of combining hand massage with pumping and showed that moms get almost 50 percent more milk when they combine pumping with hand massage. Think of this technique as moving the milk forward in your breasts, then pumping it out. Many moms also use their hands to massage while pumping or end their pump session with a few minutes of hand-expression and see dramatic results in total ounces.

**Weekly Goal #2: Bottle-Feeding**—Have you tried middle-of-the-night feed tag-teaming with your partner or support person? *Try pumping before bed, have your partner bottle-feed at the next feed (while you sleep), and you breastfeed at the following feed while your partner sleeps.* This a great way for both of you to sneak in a little more sleep. Just make sure you pay attention to your breast comfort. If you feel uncomfortably full at any time, you need to do a "comfort pump" (usually two to four minutes). Pump *just enough* to take the edge off and go back to sleep. Ignoring very full breasts or going too long at night without pumping or breastfeeding could lead to plugged ducts or mastitis.

---

### KEY ADVICE: SUPPLY

*You might have noticed when the six-week milk regulation kicked in. If you had a lot of milk, you may notice your supply settle down a bit, your breasts feel suddenly softer, leaking probably stops, baby usually drops a nighttime feed, baby's sleep gets better, and baby's stooling slows down to around once a day. Lots of changes that are all super normal.*

---

**Weekly Goal #3: Village**—Do you have friends who have babies? *Reach out and see if they'd like to meet up.* Chances are your friends have friends, and pretty soon you've got your own breastfeeding support group going!

# Week #4

**Weekly Goal #1: Pumping**—An in-the-know friend of yours with a baby probably recommended a silicone hand pump. *This week try using the silicone hand pump during one or two of your breastfeeds.* If you're fairly sure your baby will only take one breast at the feed, go ahead and attach it to the second breast. If baby is going to use both breasts at the feed, attach it to the first side when you move baby over. It's not just a "milk catcher"; the suction removes milk while baby feeds on the other side. Tip: You'll most likely get more if you use it in the morning.

> **KEY ADVICE: FUN FACT**
> *Your milk supply is on a 24-hour cycle. Most moms peak in the middle of the night, have lots of milk in the morning, and produce less and less as the day progresses.*

**Weekly Goal #2: Bottle-Feeding**—*This week, let's experiment with having another support person give a bottle.* Remember, it's *super* important that anyone who gives a bottle uses paced bottle-feeding.

**Weekly Goal #3: Village**—Finding moms to connect with can sometimes be as simple as looking in your own backyard. Research local meet-up groups and groups organized by interests. One example is Stroller Strides, a group for moms looking to exercise with baby. Not only will you make new friends, you'll also start with common interests besides your little ones.

## KEY ADVICE: GET COMFORTABLE

*Have you tried the side-lying position yet? If not, give it a try! (See "Side-Lying Hold" on page 30.) This position is great for soothing a cranky baby or "nursing down" (nursing a baby to sleep). It's also super relaxing for you. As with all bed-sharing, make sure you're following the rules for safe co-sleeping (see Sweet Sleep in the References on page 163).*

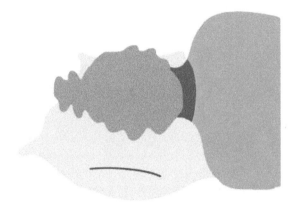

# Third Month

Okay, take a deep breath. Let's look back and appreciate how far you've come in just two short months. You learned to breastfeed, experimented with breastfeeding positions, established your milk supply, started pumping and bottle-feeding, and found your village. You've been through a *lot* these past couple of months, and you should take that in.

So now we're going to build on where we are and look at getting out, navigating sore gums, and taking the first steps in preparing for your transition back to work.

## Monthly Goal #1: Breastfeed in Public

You know those moms at restaurants who are chatting with their friends, eating lunch, scrolling through their phone, and somehow *also* managing to breastfeed their baby? Have you ever wondered how they do that? Here's the scoop: It took LOTS OF PRACTICE! Those moms and babies are advanced breastfeeders, and they put in the time to figure it out. Don't worry—you'll get there too! We'll look at small steps you can take this month to start mastering the art of public breastfeeding.

## Monthly Goal #2: Manage Sore Gums

Has your little one started to drool? Chewing on everything? Are you seeing lots of "on and off" the breast? Believe it or not, your baby's sharp teeth are cutting upward, which leads to swollen gums, and this month it may start to affect breastfeeding. We're going to look at what you can do to manage those tender gums and navigate how they change feedings.

## Monthly Goal #3: Start the Transition Back to Work

For many moms, this month is about putting a plan in place for returning to work. (If that's not you, that's okay. There are still helpful tips in this section that will help you navigate stretches away from your baby, so don't skip ahead.) It's not as daunting as it may seem, and we're going to break it down together.

# Week #1

**Weekly Goal #1: Public Breastfeeding**—When it comes to public breastfeeding, one of the most important choices you will make is what to wear. Think easy access and layers. *Look at your closet and pick out breastfeeding-friendly clothes.* Good options are button-up shirts, breastfeeding tanks with another layer on top (e.g., a big shirt or loose sweater), and shirts or other clothes made for breastfeeding moms. Try feeding in these clothes at home first and see how comfortable you are. The more you practice, the better you'll get at latching on the go, and the more confident you'll become at feeding in public spaces.

**Weekly Goal #2: Manage Sore Gums**—Even if your little one is being stoic and not complaining much, chances are their gums are hurting, *so let's get them some relief.* Common techniques for numbing gums are to offer cold or frozen teething toys, camilia (homeopathy) or herbal teething oils that provide a gentle anesthetic effect, and breastmilk popsicles (see "Teething and Biting" on page 134). Try providing relief right before the breastfeed, and see if that makes the feed more comfortable for you and your baby. As with any products you are looking at giving your baby, always check with your pediatrician to see if it's a good fit for your family.

**Weekly Goal #3: Transition Back to Work**—This is the time to start creating a little "stash" (extra milk in the freezer). The good news is you don't need a lot. Twenty to thirty ounces is the perfect amount to have in your freezer before you return to work, and most moms can collect that in two to four weeks. *This week try inserting an extra pump session in after a morning breastfeed and send that straight to the freezer.*

> **KEY ADVICE: PRO TIP**
>
> *Once you have some frozen milk, defrost a bag and check to make sure it doesn't have a funky smell. If it does, you may have an issue with excess lipase (see "Baby Rejects Frozen Milk" on page 44) or oxidation (air getting in the storage bag and causing the milk to go bad).*

## Week #2

**Weekly Goal #1: Public Breastfeeding—***This is the perfect time to reach out to a friend who has a baby and ask her to meet you.* It's even better if her baby is a little older and she's breastfeeding. Being with another mom, or a group of moms, can be very helpful when you're learning to feed in public. Have you been attending a breastfeeding support group or parenting class? Try asking someone to go out with you after the class. You'll have a chance to practice feeding in a safe and supportive environment.

**Milestone: Increased Frequency—**You may see frequency of feeds increase again this month (possibly 10 to 12 feeds every 24 hours), as those sore gums can cause more snacking. This is super normal and may come and go in waves. Hang in there.

**Weekly Goal #2: Manage Sore Gums—**This might be your baby's new favorite thing... (drumroll) ... *This week try giving them a breastmilk popsicle.* Take a silicone feeder and put chips of frozen breastmilk inside it. Hold it for your baby, running it over their gums. They will probably lick and chew it. Little do they know while they are getting a fun snack, we're sneaking in a little sore gum relief. The frozen breastmilk will help numb the gums while acting as an anti-inflammatory that helps reduce swelling.

**Weekly Goal #3: Transition Back to Work**—You may be starting to search for a caregiver to watch your baby while you're at work. *Look for a caregiver who has experience with breastmilk storage, appropriate breastmilk quantities, and paced bottle-feeding.* Ideally, once you've picked a provider to watch your baby, have them watch you bottle-feed and have them bottle-feed in front of you. Discuss breastmilk storage guidelines, how the milk will be delivered to them, and what happens if a bottle has to be thrown out.

## Week #3

**Weekly Goal #1: Public Breastfeeding**—Here's a super cool skill: *Learn to breastfeed your baby in a wrap/baby carrier.* You'll be hands-free, feeding on-the-go, and no one will have a clue what's going on in there. It does take practice, though. Look up tutorials for feeding in your carrier online, attend a baby-wearing meeting in your area, or ask a friend who has mastered it.

**Weekly Goal #2: Manage Sore Gums**—One way that babies communicate their gums are sore is by breastfeeding for a couple of minutes, then crying as they get further into the feed. Once they are past the initial let-down, they have to engage their gums more and that's when it hurts. If this crying happens, *jump in with breast massage or breast compression to speed up your milk flow (see page 33).* Baby should be much happier.

**Weekly Goal #3: Transition Back to Work**—*Reach out to your human resources department about four weeks before you return to work to let them know you're breastfeeding. Ask if there's a* *pumping room or family room available to you and, if so, how you'll reserve it and what (if any) supplies are in there. Is there a refrigerator in the room? A shared hospital-grade pump?*

**Milestone: Three-Month Growth Spurt**—Remember those growth spurts from the early weeks? They're baaaaack. This one shows up around 12 weeks and will last a few days. Don't be surprised if baby is a little cranky, gassy, and super hungry all over again.

## Week #4

**Weekly Goal #1: Public Breastfeeding**—So, you're ready to head out and try public breastfeeding—but where to go? *Try a coffee shop, park, or café with tables.* (Hint: Booths can be tricky because you can't adjust how far away you are from the table.) Avoid places where you feel like you'll have lots of eyes on you. As you grow more confident with breastfeeding in public, you'll find you can go anywhere. Before you know it, you'll be one of those moms who's a pro at multitasking while feeding.

**Weekly Goal #2: Manage Sore Gums**—*Try offering cold or frozen teething toys, especially right before feeds.* You'll need to hold the toy, but your baby should love chomping down on it and will get some gum relief from the cold.

**Weekly Goal #3: Transition Back to Work**—Before you go back to work, do a practice run where you pump and bottle-feed on the same schedule you'll follow at work. For many moms, that's 9 a.m., noon, and 3 p.m. You'll want to know ahead of time roughly how much you'll get during those work pumps.

**Milestone: Supply and Demand at Work**—We expect most babies to take a 3- to 4-ounce bottle every 3 hours while away from you. If you want to maintain a full breastmilk supply, you'll be pumping approximately every three hours at work. If you don't pump enough on your "practice run," reach out to an LC for advice on increasing supply.

## CLUSTER FEEDING

Cluster feeding means lots of frequent feeds spaced closely together. Babies often cluster feed as newborns in the late afternoon or evening and on growth spurt days. These times can be extra hard, but there are actually some important reasons babies do this.

Newborns cluster feed because they are trying to encourage your milk to transition and to establish your supply. Remember, in the first couple of weeks, babies commonly feed 10 to 12 times every 24 hours, but this settles down, and 8 times every 24 hours becomes the norm.

During growth spurts, your baby's cluster feeding helps boost your milk supply. Increased feeding frequency tells your body to send more milk. And it's pretty likely all that growing is uncomfortable for baby. We know that sucking helps lower the pain threshold in babies. Even though your baby is cueing constantly, you don't need to let them stay at the breast around the clock or give them huge bottles. If you're exhausted or sore, a pacifier or your finger (pad side–up) will go a long way toward meeting that extra suck need.

There might be another reason we see babies cluster feeding in the late afternoon and evening: Your milk is at its lowest point for the day, so babies need to do more frequent feeds to feel full. They could also be tanking up for a longer stretch of sleep at night. (Fingers crossed, right?!) Some parents place a bottle in this zone to break up all the little feeds. Babies will usually take more from a bottle at this time, which can buy you a break to eat some dinner or catch a little downtime.

# Fourth Month

**M**onth four brings lots of fun changes and a few challenges. Your baby has reached the end of the "fourth trimester." This is an age where babies often blossom and become social butterflies. That means more laughing, eye contact, and lots of social engagement. The world just became an exciting place and they are taking it *all* in! Your baby will want to be a part of the action.

## Monthly Goal #1: Manage Distracted Feeding

Keeping your baby's attention focused on breastfeeding is about to get harder and harder. Their senses are improving, and they are becoming more interested in the world around them. You'll find they now come off and look up when someone comes in the room or when they hear the TV, the neighbor's dog barking, or your phone ringing. These distractions make for lots of interrupted and shorter breastfeeding sessions. Feeding might feel less structured now. And your nipples might get sore from all the "on and off" and increased frequency. This is very normal. It's the result of your baby trying to balance feeding needs with developmental leaps and lots of stimulation in the environment.

## Monthly Goal #2: Survive the Four-Month Developmental Leap

The biggest challenge this month might be what some call the four-month sleep regression. However, it's also a developmental leap. When babies pick up new skills, their sleep may be affected at night. On top of that, there is a four-month growth spurt, distracted breastfeeding, and pre-teething. All this (often) adds up to a pretty tough two weeks. It helps to know what's happening, and we'll go over some techniques to get you through.

## Monthly Goal #3: Check In with Relationships

This is a great time to check in with people and revisit your relationships. You survived the first three months and came out the other side. Make plans with friends or reconnect with your partner. Of course, now that you have a little one, everything requires more planning, but it's worth the effort. Making sure your support system and relationships are healthy and strong is important for your mental health and for your family. So let's figure out how to make that happen.

## Week #1

**Weekly Goal #1: Distracted Feeding**—*Find a dark, quiet room for breastfeeding.* For most moms at this stage, a room with less distractions is the secret to getting a good breastfeed. You may not be able to do this for every feed, but aiming for a good focused session at least a couple of times a day may cut down on all the snacking.

**Weekly Goal #2: Developmental Leap**—The nights may be difficult for a couple of weeks. *Call in some support or tag-team with your partner to get in a good nap during the day.* Getting in some sleep will make the long, difficult nights a little more bearable.

**Weekly Goal #3: Relationship**—How are your relationships? *This is a great time to think about taking the time to relax with your partner or your friends.* Your baby's taking a bottle, so now it's possible to go out for a night and spend some couple time together if you have a partner. If date night feels like too much, think about special ways you can connect when you're together. Maybe you make plans to cook together and prepare a special meal, grab a few quiet moments to have coffee and connect in the morning, or leave a special note for the other to find.

## Week #2

**Weekly Goal #1: Distracted Feeding**—When your baby feeds, *try massaging or compressing your breast to increase the flow.* Doing so may lead to a more sustained and efficient feed. Remember to start at the top of your breast (where the milk glands are) and push the milk about halfway down your breast. You can also try compressing a full area of the breast.

**Weekly Goal #2: Developmental Leap**—If this week feels hard because sleep has been tough to come by, *focus on the positives and take note of all the cool new skills your baby has.* We know there's a link between babies learning new skills and interrupted night sleep. It should help to know that "sleep regressions" typically last a couple of weeks, and they are very normal. Your baby will return to longer stretches of sleep when this phase is over.

**Weekly Goal #3: Relationship**—Are you looking into getting a babysitter for the first time? If you don't have a local relative or close friend who would be the natural choice, ask your circle for recommendations. Another great resource can be local Girl Scouts troops. Older Girl Scouts learn CPR and infant care while earning their Cadette Babysitter Badge. Posting in local parent groups is another good way to get referrals. If you want to try the sitter out first, have them come over and watch your baby while you hang out around the house. You could also take this time to show them how you bottle-feed and care for your baby.

**Milestone: Slowing Weight Gain**—Did you know your baby's weight gain dramatically slows down at month four? Until now, your baby should have been gaining 5.5 to 8.5 ounces per week, but at month four, the rate of growth is about half that, at 3.25 to 4.5 ounces per week.

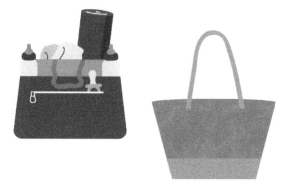

# Week #3

**Weekly Goal #1: Distracted Feeding**—*This week make sure you're offering more frequent feeds.* You might have settled into what feels like a pretty predictable pattern, but now that baby is often distracted, the feeds may have become shorter or less effective without you realizing it. If you don't actively offer more feeds, you may see it take a toll on nighttime sleep, with your baby feeding more frequently at night to get in the needed calories.

**Weekly Goal #2: Developmental Leap**—Have you revisited your baby's sleep hygiene lately? *Ramp down the stimulation in the evening, offer lots of cluster feeds, make the room as dark as possible, and try white noise.* Some families even revisit swaddling. Do what works for you and your family.

**Weekly Goal #3: Relationship**—Just getting through the day with a baby can be tough enough. It's super easy to lose sight of how responsibilities are divided up in a family. *This is a great time to sit down and make a list of what you're doing and what feels fair.* Remember that this is a season of your life, and you'll want to revisit those responsibilities and expectations periodically.

---

**KEY ADVICE: UGH! ANOTHER GROWTH SPURT**

*Don't forget the tried-and-true measures that got you through those early growth spurts. Many parents find that giving their baby gas drops with simethicone and baby-wearing are game changers, especially during growth spurts and difficult days.*

---

# *Week #4*

**Weekly Goal #1: Distracted Feeding**—Another technique to keep baby interested at the breast is to *try a different position, like the Australian Hold* (see "Australian Hold" on page 25). This position has baby straddling your leg, sitting up, and breastfeeding. Many babies can start to do it now that they have more back strength. If your baby isn't quite ready for the Australian Hold, try a modified version where they start in that position, but then you recline back so they are leaning against your torso.

**Weekly Goal #2: Developmental Leap**—Reaching the end of your rope? This is another one of those weeks where you might want to rally the troops and call in reinforcements. Having someone who can run an errand for you or tag-team so you can take a nap is invaluable. If you don't have a partner or local support, you may be able to lean on some of the new friends you made in your local breastfeeding support group or baby class. Even online mom groups sharing tips or a text from an out-of-town friend with an encouraging word will go a long way this week (see "Mom Groups Online" on page 9). *Speak up and let your support system know how to help.*

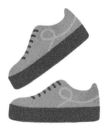

**Weekly Goal #3: Relationship—***If you're hitting a wall in your relationship, don't be afraid to call in a professional.* Many therapists offer telemedicine, which means you can meet with someone without leaving your house. Becoming parents, and the challenges that come with this transition, will naturally change your relationship. Keep the lines of communication open and figure out how you can support each other and grow together.

## BACK TO WORK

Heading back to work can trigger a lot of mixed feelings for moms. You might be feeling some anxiety and apprehension. How are you going to make it all day? Will you trust someone else to care for your baby? Will you still excel at your job while balancing your new responsibilities as a mother? Will you make enough milk? Will your baby be okay? How will you pay for childcare? On the other hand, you may be looking forward to the adult interaction and the challenges and rewards that work life brings. *It's a lot.* Talk through these feelings with a trusted friend, co-worker, or support person. Most moms will tell you that the first couple of weeks are hard, but it comes together and gets easier with time.

If possible, try to transition back to your job. Is it possible to work part-time for a few weeks? Or work from home a couple of days a week? If these options aren't available, try folding in part-time childcare a couple of weeks early, so you and your baby can ease into the new schedule. Starting midweek is another strategy that many moms use, so the first week doesn't feel quite so hard.

# Fifth Month

Ready, set, go! Month five is when you'll start to see new skills in action like rolling over, rocking, crawling and scooting. If you haven't baby-proofed your space yet, now is the time. (Tip: Get down and crawl around the room. Look at everything from baby's perspective to see what might be accessible to them.)

Most babies are doing lots of babbling by now, and you might start hearing their first attempts at speech. Get out your phone. So many cute videos ahead.

## Monthly Goal #1: Manage Older Baby Manners

Older babies can also start to pick up some *not so great* habits around feeding. Those include biting, pinching, and twiddling. OUCH. Setting clear rules and redirecting will be key, but don't worry—we'll go over specific strategies for each of these behaviors to get you through.

## Monthly Goal #2: Travel and Feed

You've also probably slipped into a nice groove as a family by this point, so maybe you're planning a family weekend away or your first family trip that involves planes and rental cars. Inevitably, the thought of travel is going to bring up concerns about feeding, feeding supplies, and equipment. Exactly how many suitcases will you need? Let's break that down with some tips and tricks and look at ways to manage breastfeeding while traveling.

## *Week #1*

**Weekly Goal #1: Manners—Biting!** This is the stage you've been dreading. How many of us have heard (or said), "I'll stop breast-feeding when my baby bites me." Good news—for most moms biting happens once or twice and sometimes not at all. *If your baby bites you, you will probably do two things instinctively: exclaim "ow!" and unlatch your baby. Both are perfect responses.* Your baby may look startled and make intense eye contact with you in an effort to gauge your reaction. Some moms will smile or laugh to make baby feel better. Doing so tells your baby that biting is a game, which you do not want to do.

Biting usually happens at the end of a feed, and to bite down a baby needs to retract their tongue first. If biting has become a problem, watch for that mouth movement and *quickly* break the latch. Also, babies often bite when they are teething, so offering gum relief remedies usually helps as well.

**Weekly Goal #2: Travel**—So, what feeding equipment or supplies do you absolutely need to bring on a trip? If you're planning to travel, make a list of the supplies you need in advance. *If you're exclusively breastfeeding, you probably just need your electric pump, a hand pump, bottles, and breastmilk storage bags or other containers.* Don't forget replacement parts for your pump, just in case. If you'll be away from refrigeration for several hours, you may want to bring a small cooler or insulated zippered lunch bag with a couple of frozen packs for milk storage. If you're also giving formula, bring a little more than you think you need in case you can't find the brand you use when you arrive. These items are the essentials. Anything you can purchase, rent, or borrow at your destination makes for lighter traveling.

Last, when traveling, don't forget to offer more breastfeeds than usual. Traveling usually means a different routine and your baby's feeding or sleep schedule may be thrown off. Frequent feeds will make for a smoother transition.

**Milestone: Demand**—Your baby may be cutting their first tooth, which will probably affect their feeding pattern. Don't be surprised if baby wants to do shorter, more frequent feeds. Try using breast massage while you feed to speed up the flow and take the pressure off your baby's gums.

# Week #2

**Weekly Goal #1: Manners**—Another breastfeeding habit that can be super irritating is when babies pinch your breast tissue or chest. Like kneading, which also happens, this behavior stimulates a faster let-down. Of course, you can keep moving baby's hand every time they pinch, but a more effective way to handle this problem is to *redirect their hand to a "nursing necklace."* Nursing necklaces are necklaces moms wear while breastfeeding. They also work well for teething babies because they are generally made of silicone and safe for baby to chew on.

**Weekly Goal #2: Travel**—Traveling by car may mean that you need to pump in the car. *Think about how you'll power your pump in a car.* Some pumps have an internal battery, which allows them to be charged and used on the go. The pumps that don't have internal batteries will usually have a car adapter accessory that's available for purchase.

Keep in mind that most pumps are strongest when plugged directly into the wall, next is plugged into the car, and last is running off an internal battery.

Other accessories that can make pumping in the car easier are hands-free pumping bras and breastmilk collection cups with tubing that attaches to most pumps. If you're not comfortable with people seeing you pump, throw on a lightweight nursing cover or use a strategically placed baby blanket.

## Week #3

**Weekly Goal #1 Manners**—Like pinching, "twiddling" is another one of those irritating habits older breastfeeding babies can pick up. Twiddling is when a baby pinches or plays with the other available nipple while feeding. It's 100 percent okay for you to set limits. You're in charge. *If your baby starts twiddling, remove their hand, make that breast inaccessible by covering it up, or redirect their hand to a nursing necklace.*

**Weekly Goal #2 Travel**—In the United States, TSA guidelines state that breastmilk and formula do not count toward your liquid allowance, and pumps are considered medical devices that don't count toward your carry-on limit. *Plan to pack your pump (if desired) and as much breastmilk or formula as you need for a plane ride.* Also bring a printout of the TSA guideline in case the TSA agent is not familiar with their policy. Think about bringing a manual hand pump too, especially if you're the only adult. You may be stuck in your seat, holding a sleeping baby and needing to pump. If you're not able to coordinate using your electric pump on the plane, a hand pump is a quick and easy way to get some breast relief.

## Week #4

**Weekly Goal: Travel**—Heading to the airport? *Consider wearing your baby instead of using a stroller.* Baby will be happy, and you'll have one less thing to lug around. If you need the stroller for the trip, consider checking it with your baggage. If you decide to bring your stroller to the gate, most airlines will have you check it as you board and you'll need to wait for it (sometimes for a while) at the gate again when you exit the plane.

As you head through security, *look for the family line.* Most airports have designated family lines to help those with small children.

If airline rules allow it and you feel baby is safe, *try to breastfeed during takeoff and landing.* Sucking stabilizes the air pressure in baby's ears and should make your baby more comfortable. If that's not an option, offer them a bottle or a pacifier or your finger (pad side–up) to suck on.

Breastfeeding throughout the flight generally equals a full and happy baby. If you need to warm up a bottle, ask the flight attendant for assistance. They will usually bring you a partially filled cup with hot water or warm it up for you.

---

**KEY ADVICE: TRAVEL TIP**

*Did you know there are companies in many cities that will rent baby supplies (strollers, cribs, high chairs, toys, etc.)? They will even deliver them to you. If you're staying in a hotel, call the concierge in advance and ask what they have at the hotel and if they can recommend any rental services. Online mom groups can also be a great resource if you're doing research on services available at your destination (see "Mom Groups Online" on page 9).*

---

## SLEEPING AND FEEDING

Sleep is a great thing for everyone. At this age, many (but not all) babies are able to sleep a longer (six- to eight-hour) stretch at night. If your baby naturally starts sleeping longer, you may notice they are squeezing in more feeds during their awake hours. Encourage your baby to feed frequently and be responsive to their cues. If you are confident your baby is getting enough calories during their awake hours but they *aren't* doing a longer stretch, it may be time to nudge them to sleep a little longer. There are many different techniques when it comes to coaching your baby. A certified pediatric sleep consultant is an invaluable asset and can help you navigate options that match your parenting style. If you don't have access to a sleep consultant, reach out to an experienced parent you trust or to one of the many groups online. If you are worried your baby is not eating enough now that they are sleeping longer, make an appointment with your pediatrician to evaluate your baby's weight and feeding pattern.

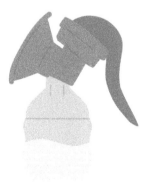

# Sixth Month

Woo hoo! Happy half-birthday! You've got six months of breastfeeding experience under your belt. This is a great time to take stock of your accomplishments and give yourself credit for how far you've come. Good job!

This month brings some big changes. We're introducing solids (see "Introducing Solid Foods" on page 106), your baby continues to become even more mobile, and we may have a few challenges crop up that can affect supply.

## Monthly Goal #1: Breastfeed Your Active Baby

An active baby is much less likely to sit still for breastfeeds. You'll start seeing a lot of breastfeeding "acrobatics," feeding from random positions, and feeding on-the-go. You might also notice that some breastfeeds are quick little check-ins more than meals. Remember that breastfeeding is more than just nutrition for your baby. It also provides a warm moment of attachment and reassurance as they start to venture out into the world.

## Monthly Goal #2: Protect Supply

Introducing solids, teething, your monthly cycle returning, and longer stretches of sleep can all affect your supply. To figure out if your output has changed, having a "test pump" to use as a reference comes in handy. Pump both breasts for 15 minutes between 6 and 9 a.m. Time it so baby hasn't breastfed for at least 90 minutes. Use that pumped volume as a reference point. If you think your supply is dipping, repeat the "test pump" and evaluate. Of course, the amount you pump is just one piece of information—and there are lots of reasons you'll get more at one pump session versus another— but it's good to have an idea of what you can typically pump at a "stand-alone" pump session in the morning.

# *Week #1*

**Weekly Goal #1: Active Baby**—A baby on-the-go is a baby who will try to breastfeed in some pretty creative positions. You'll get a foot in your mouth, an upside-down baby, or a baby who decides to roll over and take your nipple with them when they are done. (Yikes! It doesn't work like that.) Awkward feeding positions can take a toll on your nipples, quickly damaging them. *If the position is uncomfortable, unlatch baby and put them in a better position.*

**Weekly Goal #2: Protecting Supply**—As you introduce solids, pay attention to the timing of breastfeeds, or it may inadvertently affect your supply. *Always breastfeed first, then give solids.* You don't want your baby to fill up on solids and have no room for breastmilk. Breastmilk is still the main course. If you're starting with dinner as their first solid meal, try breastfeeding and then offering solids about an hour later.

**Milestone: Supply**—Introducing solids is technically the beginning of "weaning"—you're subbing out breastmilk for another food. It IS normal for your supply to start to slowly decrease over the next few months as baby's solids intake increases. The key is a slow transition. Solids under a year is mainly introduction and experimentation. Breastmilk (or formula) continues to be the main source of nutrition for your baby until they are one year old.

## Week #2

**Weekly Goal #1: Active Baby**—Have you been noticing that feeds are getting quicker and more frequent? That's very normal as your baby becomes more active and engaged in the outside world. *Just make sure you offer more frequently and encourage cluster feeding* (see "Cluster Feeding" on page 85). If you're worried your baby isn't eating enough, ask your pediatrician for a weight check.

**Weekly Goal #2: Protecting Supply**—Like a loyal friend, your pump is always there. It's easy to overlook pump maintenance. Did you know you should *change the valves, membranes, and diaphragms once a month for most pump models?* It's also a good idea to periodically re-evaluate your flange sizes. Many moms will experience their nipples getting a little larger over time from pumping and breastfeeding, and the correct flange size affects how much pumped milk you will yield, which, in turn, affects supply. Many medical insurance companies will cover pump replacement parts and supplies (like milk storage bags). Just call the customer service number for your plan and request them.

## Week #3

**Weekly Goal #1: Active Baby**—Having boundaries and rules for your baby when breastfeeding is absolutely okay (and encouraged). Your baby is going to look to you to set those rules. *If your body or your nipples are getting sore from baby's creative breast-feeding positions, go back to the basics.* Insist on good positioning and deep latch OR break the latch and postpone the feed for a later time.

Weekly Goal #2: Protecting Supply—Around this time, your baby's teething pains start to intensify. Your baby's moods (and sleep) will directly reflect the progress of those sharp little teeth making their debut. Unfortunately, that can show up as a roller coaster of emotions for your baby AND for you. It can also affect your supply because your baby isn't feeding as well. *You might need to insert a pump session or two during the day to protect your supply.*

## Week #4

Weekly Goal #1: Active Baby—Reminder: Breastfeeding isn't just about nutrition for your baby. Your active baby will want to breastfeed for emotional check-ins as they become more independent and when they get hurt, which may happen more frequently now that they are off exploring. *Continue to offer breastfeeds frequently and on demand.* Doing so not only will help protect your supply and your baby's weight gain, but also will support your baby's new active lifestyle.

Weekly Goal #2: Protecting Supply—Is everyone finally getting a long stretch of sleep at night? If so, that's great. Just watch your supply to make sure it isn't dipping and that you're not putting yourself at high risk for plugged ducts and mastitis. When your baby starts sleeping for longer stretches at night, observe your breast comfort. *If you feel uncomfortably full at any point, wake up and pump just enough to take the edge off the discomfort*—usually about two to four minutes—then go back to sleep. Pumping just a little will help keep plugged ducts at bay and will send the message to your body that it's okay to go longer between feeds at night.

## INTRODUCING SOLID FOODS

Most pediatricians recommend introducing solid foods around six months. Signs of solid readiness include good back and neck strength (baby can sit up without support), loss of the tongue-thrust reflex (tongue extends even when lips are touching), ability to pinch and hold things, and an increased interest in solids. (Is your baby watching every bite you take?)

Popular first foods include applesauce and smashed avocados, bananas, and sweet potatoes. Make sure you space out new foods by two to three days so if there's an allergic reaction you'll know what caused it. Allergic reactions or sensitivities to foods can show up as rashes on the body, a diaper rash, wheezing or difficulty breathing, excessive spitting up, or gastrointestinal discomfort.

The idea of offering chunkier foods at six months (versus purees), letting babies feed themselves, and following the baby's lead is called "baby-led weaning." Start with pieces of food the baby can hold and bite into—spear or wedge shapes work best.

Start by offering one meal a day, and slowly work up to three meals and two snacks by one year. Continue to follow your baby's cues and breastfeed on demand. Solids will *slowly* replace calories previously provided by nursing, but even at 12 months, babies are still getting most of their calories from breastmilk.

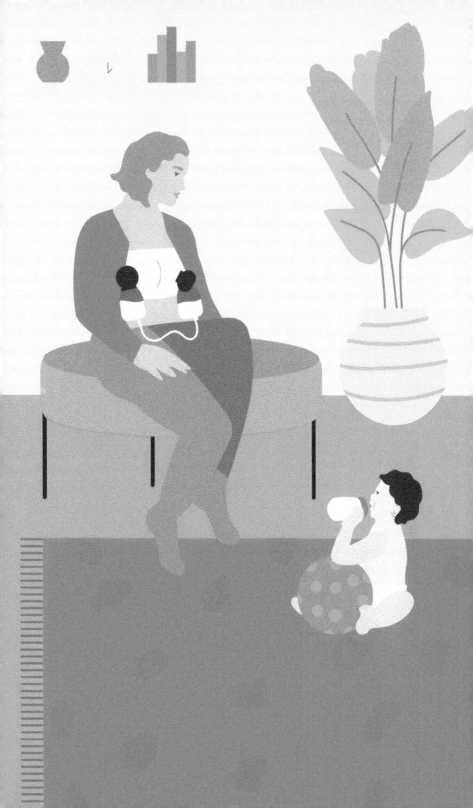

# PART THREE

# Months 7 to 12

## Seventh Month

Can you believe how much your baby has changed over the past few months? Now you have an active, engaged baby who is breastfeeding *and* eating solids. Remember those early days when you struggled to latch your baby, the nights were long, and every day felt like one endless growth spurt? Now you're a pro! Be sure to support the new breastfeeding moms you see out in the world. Remember: They are watching you and wondering how you make it look so easy.

Having said that, we can still have little hiccups that pop up in these next six months. Sometimes getting breastfeeding advice at this age can be even harder because you're probably not attending a breastfeeding support group or talking to your LC much anymore. (Tip: Both can offer a lot of support for these months too. If you're struggling with an issue, pull out that number and give your LC a ring! Or reach out to moms in your support group for some sage wisdom.)

## Monthly Goal #1:
## Avoid Sore Nipples (Not Again!)

Earlier we talked about all those sneaky culprits that can lead to sore nipples—teething, distracted breastfeeding, and baby acrobatics. You'll see those continue over the next several weeks with a few new ones we'll look at this month.

Any time your nipples are sore (for *whatever* reason), you're going to want to fold in some relief measures. Remember that your own expressed breastmilk is a great healing measure. Frequently express a few drops of breastmilk to dab on your nipples. (Frequently means every 15 minutes, or as often as you think of it.) You can also order a fresh pack of hydrogel pads or give your nipples a break by subbing out a few breastfeeding sessions for pumping and bottle-feeding. In more extreme cases, you might want to try all-purpose nipple ointment (APNO), a prescription nipple cream that your OB/Gyn can prescribe for you when needed.

## Monthly Goal #2: Build on Solids

You probably introduced solids last month and have been having a ton of fun watching your baby explore this new culinary world. (By the way, if your baby isn't into solids yet, don't worry. Many babies take a little longer to embrace them. Keep offering and follow your baby's lead.)

As we head into this month, you're probably offering one meal a day. Did you know you can vary when that meal is offered? Some days it may be breakfast, whereas on another day, dinner is what's on the menu. No matter which meal you choose, it's super important to eat with your baby when you can. Modeling is one of the main ways babies learn, so let them see you eat.

## *Week #1*

**Weekly Goal #1: Sore Nipples**—Did you recently discover a new rash in the shape of your baby's mouth on your breast? The culprit could be solids. *Pay attention to any new rashes that pop up on your breast when you introduce solids.* Some moms develop eczema when solids in the baby's mouth make contact with their breast. If that happens, see a dermatologist for treatment. Avoid breastfeeding right after offering solids, or gently wiping your breast off with a wet washcloth right after feeding may help.

**Weekly Goal #2: Building on Solids**—*Let your baby decide what and how much solid food they eat.* Don't make mealtimes a war. Don't force food when they're turning their heads away or pressure them into taking "just one more bite." Babies are great self-regulators and you want to encourage this behavior. And you do have some control. You get to decide what you offer, and how frequently you offer it. Respecting your baby's cues when it comes to solids lays the foundation for healthy eating habits.

*"The American Academy of Pediatrics recommends breastfeeding for six months."* **Nope!** *It's easy to see where the confusion crops up because the wording is confusing. Here's what their recommendation actually says:*

*"The American Academy of Pediatrics believes that breastfeeding is the optimal source of nutrition through the first year of life. We recommend exclusively breastfeeding for about the first six months of a baby's life, and then gradually adding solid foods while continuing breastfeeding until at least the baby's first birthday. Thereafter, breastfeeding can be continued for as long as both mother and baby desire it."*

*Let's break that down. The ideal is to give your baby breastmilk exclusively for 6 months, breastmilk plus solids from (approximately) 6 months to 12 months, and breastmilk and solids beyond 12 months as long as mom and baby wish to keep going. That's different than what you usually hear, right? Spread the word!*

**Weekly Goal #1: Sore Nipples**—Has pumping become more and more uncomfortable over the past few months? *Reassess your flanges to make sure they are still a good fit.* Breastfeeding and pumping will often cause your nipples to get larger over time. That means the flange that fit well at three months may not be a good fit anymore. And a flange that's too small can lead to sore nipples!

When you assess each flange, look at how your nipple fits in the tunnel at the end of the feeding. You should see the pump pulling your nipple, a little bit of the areola going into the tunnel, and the nipple moving freely. If your nipple fills up the tunnel and rubs against the sides, the flange size is too small. Try a larger size and see if it feels better. (Fun fact: The correct flange size will not only feel better, but you'll also probably yield more milk at each pump session.)

---

**KEY ADVICE: FUN FACT**

*Human bodies are not symmetrical. You may have two different-size nipples and need to use different flange sizes. Super common! Experiment with larger (or smaller) flange sizes to see what the best fit is for you. The "right" size is the one that feels most comfortable.*

---

**Weekly Goal #2: Building on Solids**—It's so easy to get caught up in the excitement of offering solids to your baby, but ramping up too fast (either the size of the meal or the number of meals per day) can affect your milk supply and your baby's comfort. *Take it slowly, gradually increase volume and frequency, and follow your baby's lead.*

At this stage, each meal of solids should be about two table-spoons and you should be offering one meal a day. Over the next six months, you'll gradually add more and more solids into your baby's routine—until you're at three meals and two snacks by 12 months. Take your time. Solids can be constipating, so too much too fast can lead to tummy troubles and slower stooling.

## Week #3

**Weekly Goal: Sore Nipples**—When moms see lower pump volumes, they sometimes respond by turning up the vacuum (suction) to compensate. *Check that your pump vacuum is at the highest comfortable setting for you but not higher or you'll get sore!* In fact, if you're in pain, your brain inhibits let-down, which works against you.

Have you seen a crack form at the base of your nipple? That's classic pump damage and a sign that you've got the suction up too high.

If you do see your milk supply decreasing quickly, instead of turning up the pump suction, take a look at frequency of and efficacy of milk removal. That's always the main factor in deter-mining your milk supply.

**Milestone: The Gains**—Using the World Health Organization (WHO) Child Growth Standards—what we base all our growth charts on—the average weight gain for babies 6 to 12 months is 1.75 to 2.75 ounces per week. That's a dramatic slow-down from earlier weight gain.

## Week #4

**Weekly Goal: Balancing Solids and Breastfeeding**—Solids can be constipating for babies, and this can be problematic on a few fronts. The AAP says a baby is constipated "if stools are hard, dry and painful to pass." Struggling to move stools, having several days between stools, or seeing a tummy that's hard can also be signs. *Pay close attention to how foods affect your baby by keeping a food diary.* Although every baby is different, some foods are more constipating than others. Watch to see how bananas, carrots, cheese, pasta, and potatoes affect your little one.

# CONSTIPATION

Is baby constipated? Certain foods and a too-fast increase in solids both cause constipation, which can also occur with an increase in formula or the introduction of a new formula. You might have noticed that your little one might not be feeling as hungry because they are backed up, which can affect feeding and weight gain.

For all these reasons, it's important to let your pediatrician know what's going on. Your pediatrician may recommend giving apple, pear, or prune juice, or an infant suppository. In addition to folding in the "p" foods (peaches, pears, peas, plums, and prunes) to baby's meals, try a bath followed by tummy massage. When baby is relaxed, apply some unscented (or gentle) lotion to your hands and apply clockwise circular strokes to baby's tummy. YouTube has great infant massage resources, including some for digestion and constipation. Massage should be relaxing for your baby. They get a spa treatment and you might see some bowel movement.

Have you been storing breastmilk in a deep freezer? (Breastmilk is good for 6 to 12 months in a deep freezer.) If so, do you happen to have some breastmilk from the first few weeks? This would be a *great* time to defrost it, because that frozen breastmilk contains colostrum, which is a natural laxative! Who knew, right?

Some families also find giving an infant probiotic helpful. Always ask your pediatrician about introducing new products, even those that are sold over the counter.

# Eighth Month

Your eight-month-old is probably feeling super curious, actively exploring the world, and adding new skills by the day—such a fun stage! But where do we find time for feeding in that busy schedule?

## Monthly Goal #1: Feed a Busy Baby

We're going to have to get creative and tackle this one head on. A lot of busy babies will naturally move some of their feeding to nighttime, which can make nights harder for both of you. Another unintended consequence might be slower than expected weight gain. If in doubt, always check in with your pediatrician to find out if your baby is gaining well.

Even though we may not be able to completely avoid the struggles that come with feeding a busy baby, we're going to look at ways to be proactive and get those daytime feeds in.

## Monthly Goal #2: Manage Nursing Strikes

Another very common breastfeeding challenge at this time is a nursing strike. (Ugh.) Here's the most important thing I want you to know about nursing strikes: They are super common, and they don't mean it's the end of breastfeeding.

When a nursing strike happens, take a deep breath and keep these two big goals for survival in mind:

Feed your baby. We have to keep baby fed, even if it means more pumping and bottle-feeding.

Protect your supply. If baby is getting more bottles, you need to pump to replace that milk and tell your body that a feed happened. I know it's much easier to pull a bag out of your stash without replacing it, but you'll start to see a dip in your breastmilk supply if you do so. We're going to look at proactive steps you can take this month to help prevent nursing strikes. For tips on how to deal with a nursing strike when it happens, see "Nursing Strike Action Plan" on page 122.

## *Week #1*

Weekly Goal #1: Feeding a Busy Baby—If baby is on the go during the day, *let's look at creating a routine and offering breastfeeds at times they are more willing to settle in for a good feed.* Try scheduling a daily walk and breastfeeding as soon as you get home. The outside air and all the stimulation that goes with a walk is magic, and you'll come home with a sleepy baby who is willing to snuggle and feed well. Many moms find that mornings and late afternoons are the best times for these daily walks.

**Weekly Goal #2**: Nursing Strike—*Have you folded in a daily routine for gum relief? If not, now's the time!* (See "Teething and Biting" on page 134.) Many parents don't think about offering gum relief measures unless baby complains or makes their discomfort very obvious. Proactively treating gums can help prevent nursing strikes that result from sore gums.

Often a nursing strike—or at least receiving mixed, confusing feeding cues at the breast—is the first sign that a baby's gums are bothering them. Other signs can be drooling, chewing on their hands, and putting everything in their mouth. You may see that baby does okay for the first few minutes (hello, first let-down), then comes off crying when it's time for them to engage their mouth more.

**Milestone: The Demand**—We're still expecting baby to feed approximately the same number of times every 24 hours. Depending on how your baby is doing with solids, though, you may see one of the feeds being slowly replaced by a solid-food meal.

## Week #2

**Weekly Goal #1**: Feeding a Busy Baby—*If you haven't mastered public breastfeeding yet, this week is a great time to work on that skill.* You're likely finding that you're out and about with your baby much more often now, so feeding on the go is pretty essential for you and your busy baby. Try taking small steps. If you're in a mall, look for a lounge in a big department store or an empty corner of the food court. Meet up with one or two friends for an early or late lunch, when you know the restaurant will be less crowded. Find a La Leche League meeting in your neighborhood, and practice public breastfeeding surrounded by the comfort of other breastfeeding moms. A nice thing about La Leche League meetings is you'll see babies of all ages there—tiny babies to toddlers. And you might make new friends as well, which is always a bonus.

**Weekly Goal #2: Nursing Strike**—*Keep an eye on your supply!* Has your supply been dipping? Sometimes babies will start to lose interest in breastfeeding when there's less "payoff" at the breast. Have you done a "test pump" lately? (See the sixth month "Monthly Goal #2: Protect Supply" on page 102.) Inserting an extra pump or two per day can be a quick way to get a supply boost.

## Week #3

**Weekly Goal #1: Feeding a Busy Baby**—A sleepy baby is usually receptive to breastfeeding. If your baby is resisting feeds during the day, catching those longer sleepy feeds right before or after naps might be the secret to getting more daytime feeds in. *If you aren't already, try side-lying with your baby and "nursing down" to sleep.* (See "Side-Lying Hold" on page 30.) Side-lying is a super ergonomic position that's comfortable for you *and* for baby. It's also cozy and works like a charm for getting a cranky baby to sleep.

**Weekly Goal #2: Nursing Strike**—A nursing strike (especially if it's on one side only) might be an early sign of a plugged duct. Having a plug usually slows the flow, and babies can react by losing interest. *Stay in touch with your breasts. Regularly feel for hard or tender areas, and be on the lookout for longer stretches of time where you're not breastfeeding or pumping.* Big changes to your feeding schedule can lead to plugged ducts.

## Week #4

**Weekly Goal: Feeding a Busy Baby**—*Don't forget about breast-feeding in your baby carrier.* When your baby was little, you might have spent some time feeding in your soft carrier or baby wrap. Now you're most likely using a sturdier "structured" carrier when you leave the house. Learning to breastfeed while wearing this type of carrier is worth your time and effort. You'll be feeding hands-free, which is super convenient. Imagine the places you can go while feeding—grocery store, restaurant, errands, maybe even work. Give it a try at home, especially when baby doesn't want to take a break from playing, is having a cranky moment, or is in the cluster feeding portion of the evening.

Learning *how* to feed in your carrier is the tricky part. Every wrap requires a different technique or hold, so start with the manufacturer's website. It often has great tutorial videos. Look on YouTube and social media next. Baby-wearing friends are another valuable resource. And don't forget about local baby-wearing groups or baby-wearing instructors.

---

**KEY ADVICE: MYTH BUSTER**

*"There's no benefit to breastfeeding once you're giving formula." Nope! Some breastmilk is always better than no breastmilk. It absolutely does not have to be all or nothing. Many families choose to combo-feed with breastmilk and formula. You should do what's right for you and your family. Every family is different. And there's NO SHAME in whatever you decide.*

---

# NURSING STRIKE ACTION PLAN

Nursing strikes happen, even when you're doing everything "right." If your baby strikes, know that it's temporary. This is not your baby weaning. Here are some techniques for getting your baby back to breast:

1. **Don't make breastfeeding a battle.** If you push too hard, your baby will become breast averse and won't like going there. Keep your offers quick and low stress.

2. **Keep offering and offer frequently.** Don't give up. Offer many times each day.

3. **Offer gum relief measures.** It could be those pesky sore gums. Let's offer some relief, especially right before feeds, and see if that helps.

4. **Squeeze in "sneaky feeds."** Feed in a dark room, as a snack between feeds, and when baby is sleepy (falling asleep or just waking up).

5. **Evaluate your supply.** Could lower supply be the culprit? Use breast massage or compressions to speed up flow and work in ways of increasing supply, if needed.

6. **Look for signs of cold or illness in your baby.** A stuffy nose, an ear infection, an upset tummy, or constipation can make your baby not want to feed. Rule out anything that might be causing them to feel unwell.

7.  **Change positions.** Switching up breastfeeding positions is the equivalent of turning your computer on and off.
Sometimes it just works.

8.  **Add motion.** Walking and feeding or feeding while bounc-
ing on a yoga ball might also be the magic bullet.

Try these tips. Switch them up. And keep trying them. If you're
persistent, your baby will come back to the breast, usually within a
week or two. In the meantime, you need to feed the baby and protect
your supply. Hang in there!

# Ninth Month

Your baby is getting bigger! Month nine brings a little one who is working on moving and communicating—crawling, cruising, nodding, shaking their head no, and exerting some independence. This month you're in for lots of personality and great photo ops.

On the feeding front, teething will now be on your radar (on and off) for quite a while. You'll be gradually increasing solids. By now you may have introduced a second daily meal, and you should be gradually increasing the complexity of the solids. Think shredded soft cheese instead of just smashed sweet potatoes and avocados.

And although breastfeeding is easy in many ways now, moms of babies this age can start worrying about how effective breast-feeds are as they start to see lots of "poky feeding" and sleeping at the breast. We'll look at managing this new stage and see what's going on.

Along with those changes, you might have started to notice changes in your body. Does it feel like your monthly cycle is returning? We're going to take a look at how that impacts breastfeeding and some tips for balancing breastfeeding and the return of menstruation.

## Monthly Goal #1: Manage the Return of Your Monthly Cycle

Let's start by looking at the numbers. Thirty-seven percent of breastfeeding moms see the return of menstruation at 6 to 12 months, whereas 48 percent see it return between 12 and 24 months. A few months before your cycle *officially* returns, you'll probably feel like it's *about* to return. Full and tender breasts? Check. Crampy? Check. Mood swings? Check, check, check. But it's a no-show. Your hormones are fluctuating and your body is getting ready to return to menstruation. Unfortunately, it's also common to see a monthly dip in your supply and to experience sore nipples from the hormones.

## Monthly Goal #2: Adjust for Sleepy Feeds

Remember the days when your baby was a marathon feeder? Now we have the opposite issue. Your baby goes to breast, does a quick little feed, then wants to hang out or sleep. It'll probably have you wondering if they are actually feeding and if there's a problem. The short answer is it's probably normal. But it can also be something to watch. We'll troubleshoot this issue and make sure a larger problem is not developing.

## *Week #1*

**Weekly Goal #1: Cycle Returning**—If your monthly cycle has returned, you've probably noticed a dip in your supply each month for a few days around ovulation. *Many moms find that taking a combination supplement of calcium and magnesium helps take the edge off the dip.* The recommended calcium daily dosage on KellyMom.com is "between 500 mg calcium/250 mg magnesium and 1500 mg calcium/750 mg magnesium (the higher dosage is generally more effective)." Big calcium supplements should not be taken by themselves because the body won't absorb the nutrient efficiently. Instead, they should be part of a calcium and magnesium (or calcium, magnesium, and zinc) combo.

The amount of supplement depends on what you're eating—the more meat you eat usually means the more calcium and magnesium you're getting. If you are not a vegetarian or vegan, the lower dosage may do the trick. If you need to supplement more than 500 milligrams of calcium per day, split it up so you're not taking this dosage all at once—absorption works better when you take no more than 500 milligrams at one time.

Weekly Goal #2: Sleepy Feeds—Remember that breastfeeding also meets your baby's emotional needs and the need for physical touch. Now that your baby is more active, some of these quick feeds might be "check-ins" with you. *Embrace the check-in and savor baby's snuggles.* As long as your baby is gaining weight appropriately, you can feel confident they are getting enough calories between breastfeedings and solids.

## *Week #2*

Weekly Goal #1: Cycle Returning—If the monthly dip in your cycle is so severe that your baby often seems hungry and not satiated, you may want to *do a few extra pump sessions the other three weeks of the month.* The extra pumping will give you more of a stash to draw from when you need it, and the extra milk removal will probably boost your supply. If using your double electric pump seems like too much work, consider using your silicone hand pump a few sessions a week for extra milk.

Weekly Goal #2: Sleepy Feeds—What looks like "poky" or ineffi-cient feeds might just be your baby becoming a better feeder. It's super normal for babies to get faster and more efficient at feeding as they get older. *Observe your baby's body language after feeds.* If they seem full, happy, and satiated after a feed and your breast feels softer, chances are the feed was exactly what your baby needed. No need to worry.

## Week #3

**Weekly Goal: Cycle Returning**—Fluctuating hormones may also cause your nipples to be more tender during ovulation. *Try experimenting with different breastfeeding positions to see if you can find one that's more comfortable.* If that doesn't work, try swapping out a breastfeed or two for pumping and bottle-feeding because the pump is usually less aggressive on your nipples.

**Milestone: The Demand**—You'll probably see another growth spurt the first week of month nine, which means a baby who is feeding more frequently (back to 10 to 12 times every 24 hours) and is gassy, cranky, and waking up more at night. This spurt should last a few days to a week. You've got this!

## Week #4

**Weekly Goal: Sleepy Feeds**—Breastfeeds are also great first aid. If your baby is coming to you after a fall or a hard time, a breastfeed instantly makes everything better. It may not be nutrition your baby needs in that moment. *Embrace the calming effect of breastfeeding. It's your superpower.* In fact, there have been many studies that confirm breastfeeding's protective effect on infant pain levels.

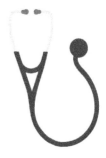

## BURNOUT

By now you've been breastfeeding for as long as you were pregnant. Starting to feel a bit of burnout at this stage is very common. Some good advice is never quit on a bad day. You may have a different opinion in a few days. And you're so close to the one-year mark!

This is also an important time to turn to your village for support. Reach out to fellow moms who've experienced the same thing, write a long post on a forum, or talk to someone close to you about the pressures and stresses you're feeling right now.

It's also okay to re-evaluate your breastfeeding goals. *Breastfeeding should work in your life.* Instead of completely weaning, consider partial weaning and reducing the amount of pumping or breastfeeding you're doing. There's a plan that's going to feel right.

# Tenth Month

Let's focus on YOU this month. Have you been finding time for self-care? Remember that you're an integral part of this feeding system, and you have to take care of yourself. Let's examine the ways you can take care of yourself while balancing feeding and caring for your baby.

## Monthly Goal #1: Focus on You

Life with a busy baby can be hectic. It's easy to focus on all you need to do and not prioritize making time for yourself. Ask friends and family for support, so you can do something for yourself. You'll be happier and healthier for making the effort.

## Monthly Goal #2: Check Your Supply

It's common for some moms to feel a slight dip in their milk supply this month. A small dip is expected as we continue to increase solids. (You should be offering two meals at this point, and possibly a third.) Protecting your supply in these later months and ensuring it stays in the appropriate zone will help you reach your breastfeeding goals.

### Week #1

**Weekly Goal #1: Focus on You**—This is about the time many moms start looking at exercise and weight loss. Both are compatible with breastfeeding *as long as your weight loss doesn't exceed two pounds a week*. More than that can affect your breastmilk supply.

When exercising, try to pump or breastfeed right before (for breast comfort) and wear a supportive sports bra. Watch out for exercise that involves repetitive arm movements, which can cause plugged ducts in some women. You may also find that baby doesn't want to breastfeed after you exercise because of the salt on your skin. If so, take a quick shower before feeding.

**Weekly Goal #2: Supply Check**—Have you done a test pump lately? (See the sixth month "Monthly Goal #2: Protect Supply" on page 102.) This is a great way to see how much your supply has changed over the past few months. It would be normal to see about a 20 percent decrease in your pumped volume at this point (compared to where you were before you introduced solids). If you see more than that, *try inserting a pump session after a breastfeed each day for a couple of weeks, then repeat the test pump.* You should see a little boost.

## Week #2

**Weekly Goal #1: Focus on You**—Take a moment to look at your relationships with your partner, family, and friends. *Focus on one of those relationships this week and identify two to three ways you can work on strengthening it.* Perhaps you can meet a friend for lunch or set aside some time to really connect with your partner.

**Weekly Goal #2: Supply Check**—*This week let's do a pump check.* Have you been replacing your valves and membranes each month? Are your flanges still the right fit? (It's normal for your nipples to grow larger over time, which would require a larger flange size.) Not keeping up on pump part maintenance can lead to your pump not removing milk as well as it should. And *that* can lead to a dip in supply.

## Week #3

**Weekly Goal: Focus on You**—What makes you feel like your old self? Is it a hobby you put down many months ago? Or time you devote to a cause? Maybe it's making a particular meal? Sneaking away to catch a matinee by yourself (or with a friend)? *This week focus on doing something that makes you feel like your old self.* Doing so will increase your energy and lend balance to your life.

**Milestone: Growth Charts**—How important is the growth chart? Well, your pediatrician should be using the WHO Child Growth Standards. These standards are a valuable tool but only one piece of the picture. Pediatricians will typically look at the *trend* of weight gain to see if your baby is roughly "staying on their curve" or "in their bracket." A baby trending downward in weight brackets can be a sign that your doctor needs to take a closer look at what's going on.

## *Week #4*

**Weekly Goal: Supply Check**—Still need a little boost to your supply? *Revisit having oatmeal for breakfast in the morning or including brewer's yeast in your diet.* (Brewer's yeast capsules rather than the granules tend to work better for most moms.) Although more research is needed, anecdotal evidence supports taking these supplements to increase supply.

---

**KEY ADVICE: FUN FACT**

*Moms often report record-breaking pump volumes after a massage, so book one ASAP! If you don't have the time or resources for a professional massage, ask your partner or a friend to give you a shoulder rub. It will also work wonders. Moms often don't realize how much time they spend looking down at their little one while they breastfeed. This causes tension to build up in their body over time, which takes a toll. At the very least, get into the habit of taking a break during feeds to look away from your baby and roll out your neck and shoulders. Your body will thank you.*

---

# TEETHING AND BITING

By now your baby probably has a tooth or two and is actively teething. When your baby has a tooth coming in, life may feel like a rollercoaster. You'll see a cranky baby with faster or more frequent feeds and a lot more night-waking. But as soon as that tooth pops out, you'll both get instant relief. (Yay, happy baby!)

Let's look at how teething affects breastfeeding:

**Shorter Feeds.** Those gums hurt (*a lot*), so your baby is going to do shorter feeds. This means a less structured feeding schedule for you and possibly more nighttime feeds.

**Uncomfortable Baby during Feeds.** Does your baby do okay the first few minutes but come off and start crying? Sore gums are to blame again. Try using breast massage or compressions to get more milk flowing.

**Biting.** Be on the lookout for baby retracting their tongue at the end of the feed, and be ready to quickly break the latch!

**Sore Nipples.** Make sure you're frequently dabbing drops of expressed breastmilk on your nipples and using hydrogels if needed. Also, try switching breastfeeding positions, which should also give your nipples some relief.

Camilia (homeopathy), herbal teething oils, cold or frozen teething toys, and breastmilk popsicles are popular teething relief measures. As with any product, check with your pediatrician before trying something new, including over-the-counter products and medicines like ibuprofen.

# Eleventh Month

Did this year fly by? Has it been easier or harder than you thought it would be? Probably both, right? Yet somehow we're at month 11 and it's almost your little one's birthday!

Have you thought about how you'll celebrate? Some families plan a big celebration for baby with super cute smash cake photos, whereas others gather family and friends, bring in great food, open a bottle of wine, and celebrate getting to this milestone together. Do what feels special for you and your family.

And what does this month mean for feeding? Are you ready to wrap it up? Or are you on a roll and excited about keeping a good thing going? (You can also be somewhere in between and that's absolutely okay.) Weaning or continuing to breastfeed beyond a year is a personal and sometimes complicated decision.

Maybe you're not ready to wean, but you want to tweak your breastfeeding relationship with your child.

Let's explore both weaning and setting limits around breastfeeding this month.

## Monthly Goal #1: Wean

There are several ways (or styles) of going about weaning.

**Quick weaning** is the fastest way. It usually takes a couple of weeks and is used for emergency situations where it's necessary to wean as fast as possible. The slower the wean, the easier it is for you and baby.

**Transitional weaning** takes anywhere from four to eight weeks and involves a transition from one feeding plan to another.

**Child-led weaning** follows the child's lead and is usually the slowest approach to weaning by gradually dropping one breastfeed or pump session at a time.

***Whatever you do, don't stop cold turkey!*** Weaning too fast can lead to plugged ducts and mastitis. If you're not sure how to wean, an LC is a great resource and will help you come up with a personalized plan. If connecting with an LC isn't an option, try dropping one breastfeed or pump session at a time.

## Monthly Goal #2: Set Boundaries around Breastfeeding

Older babies will often exert their newfound independence. The good news is you're still in charge and get to create the boundaries that feel good to you.

It's okay to say no, not here, and not right now. *Establish boundaries with breastfeeding to make it work for you.* Your baby is old enough to start to understand your tone of voice and new patterns and can delay a feed when needed. A one-year-old who is very busy during the day may want to breastfeed throughout the night. This schedule might work for baby, but mom ends up getting no rest. It's okay to tell your baby, "We only breastfeed when the sun is out," or, "We don't breastfeed in bed." As with all boundaries, consistency is very important.

### Week #1

**Weekly Goal #1: Weaning**—Many moms choose a transitional weaning plan that *drops one or two breastfeeds or pump sessions per week.* Typically, you do that by converting the breastfeed to a pump and pumping a few minutes less each day, or by skipping the breastfeed altogether and pumping for comfort when needed. Of course, baby still needs to be fed. If your baby is under a year, formula replaces breastmilk. If your baby is over a year, you can increase solids to compensate for the dropped feed.

Weekly Goal #2: Setting Boundaries—Have you reached the stage at which your baby is coming over and lifting your shirt to breastfeed? If that's fine with you, no need to change anything. But if it's not okay, you can let your baby know in a clear and calm voice that it's not okay and redirect them. *Teach your child how to ask for a breastfeed in a way that's comfortable to you.* Some moms teach their baby to use the word "milk" in American Sign Language (a one-handed sign, squeezing your hand—like milking a cow).

---

**KEY ADVICE: MYTH BUSTER**

*"The longer you wait to wean, the harder it's going to be."* Incorrect! *How your child reacts to weaning is much more dependent on their personality and how ready they are to wean than on the number of months they breastfed. The same goes for you, too, because it can be hard to say goodbye to this extraordinary time of bonding and development.*

---

## Week #2

Weekly Goal #1: Weaning—When you're weaning, paying attention to how comfortable your breasts feel is very important. You're at a higher risk for plugged ducts and mastitis now. Regardless of the technique you're using, *do a comfort pump or hand express if your breasts are uncomfortably full.* Some moms also find it helpful to take sunflower lecithin during weaning to help ensure against plugged ducts. Lecithin makes breastmilk less viscous (thick and sticky) and less likely to cause plugs.

**Weekly Goal #2: Setting Boundaries**—You're in charge of where you feed. *If you prefer not to feed in public or at a specific location, let your child know and give them something else to eat.* Be sure to pay attention to your breasts and avoid going too long without feeding or pumping—you don't want to end up with a plugged duct.

## BIRTH CONTROL

Birth control can affect your milk supply, so make sure you let your OB/Gyn know you're breastfeeding. In general, if you're taking an oral contraceptive, you want to avoid one with estrogen. They can come in several forms, including the combination birth control pill, skin patch, and vaginal ring. Safer options for your milk supply include progestin-only pill (also called the "mini-pill"), progestin-releasing IUDs (Mirena, Skyla), the birth control injection (Depo-Provera), and birth control implant (Implanon, Nexplanon). The safest options for your milk supply are contraceptives that don't contain hormones. Any birth control that contains hormones can affect your supply, so talk to your OB/Gyn about the appropriate contraption and dosage for you.

## Week #3

**Weekly Goal #1: Weaning**—Weaning causes your hormones to fluctuate and can lead to mood swings (just like in the early days of pregnancy). *Be on the lookout for mood swings and recognize* *they are a part of the process of weaning and should be tem-porary.* Weaning may also trigger postpartum depression and postpartum anxiety, or both. If you are not feeling like yourself, reach out to a counselor or therapist or call the Postpartum Support International at 1-800-944-4773 for help in English or Spanish or go to Postpartum.net.

**Weekly Goal #2: Setting Boundaries**—You also get to *decide what word you use for breastfeeding.* Sometimes a word gets assigned for breastfeeding (like "milky" or "mommy milk"), and it may not be one you're fond of or want your child saying in public. This is the time to change it if you'd like. Your new word can be anything that feels good to you.

## *Week #4*

**Weekly Goal: Weaning**—The conclusion of breastfeeding is almost always emotional for moms. It's the end of a special stage in your relationship with your baby. *Many moms find it meaningful to mark the moment by doing something special to commemorate the end of the journey.* You could write a letter to your baby and share your feelings, go out on the town for a night with friends, take a picture of the last breastfeed, put a handwrit-ten note on the last bag of frozen milk, order a piece of breastmilk jewelry for yourself, or create an announcement on social media that you're done (see "How Weaning Will Affect You" on page 157).

## BREASTFEEDING AND PREGNANCY

Are you pregnant? Did you notice your supply suddenly dip? Pregnancy typically leads to a decrease in milk supply. That may or may not be okay with you depending on where you are in your weaning plans. *Try increasing solids or feed solids before the breast-feed so baby ends up full and satiated.*

Another early sign of pregnancy is sore nipples. The usual tools for nipples that hurt (breastmilk, hydrogels) are less likely to work because the cause is hormones. *Try switching breastfeeding positions or subbing out some breastfeeding for pumping, which should be gentler on your nipples. When you're pumping, you may find you need to use a lower vacuum setting.* Go as low as you need to go, mama.

Nausea and morning sickness while breastfeeding can go either way. Although most moms find morning sickness to be much less intense when breastfeeding, some get nauseated with every let-down. *Try playing with breastfeeding positions as well as when and how long baby feeds to see if any of these factors make a difference in the intensity of your nausea.*

# Twelfth Month

Confetti! Balloons! Pop the Champagne and cue the marching band! YOU DID IT!

You breastfed your baby for a year! You met the AAP's recommendation! If you're like most moms, you had many struggles and many wins along the way—high moments and low moments. But you got here. You should feel *very proud*. Breastfeeding for a year is a huge accomplishment. According to the CDC, as of 2016 only 36 percent of American babies were still receiving breastmilk at 12 months. It's a *very real* struggle for families to receive the support they need to meet their breastfeeding goals. The good news is the percentages are increasing and we're heading in the right direction.

Now that we're here, what's next? We talked about weaning last month, so this month let's talk about breastfeeding your toddler. Many moms decide to keep going at this point.

## Monthly Goal #1: Breastfeed a Toddler

Why should you continue breastfeeding? Remember, breastmilk is *always* beneficial for your baby. Unfortunately, not much research has been done on children who breastfeed past the age of two, but according to KellyMom.com, "the available information indicates that breastfeeding continues to be a valuable source of nutrition and disease protection for as long as breastfeeding continues."

## Monthly Goal #2: Handle Criticism

Does everyone suddenly seem to have an opinion about how you feed your baby? Moms who breastfeed past age one in the United States are often subject to lots of opinions about "extended" breastfeeding. There are many ways to deal with unwelcome advice and opinions, and we'll review some suggestions in this chapter.

## *Week #1*

Weekly Goal #1: Breastfeeding a Toddler—Parents are often surprised how the timing and frequency of breastfeeds shift as the child gets older (see "Toddler Breastfeeding Schedule" on page 153). Contrary to stereotypes, breastfeeding toddlers also eat solids and don't spend large chunks of time breastfeeding. Breastfeeds tend to be quick check-ins, often before bed or right after waking up. *Embrace this new schedule.* You should find it much easier than the early days!

Weekly Goal #2: Handling Criticism—If a partner, loved one, or friend is genuinely curious about why you are breastfeeding your toddler, use their questions as an opportunity to educate. There are lots of great resources available at websites such as KellyMom.com, La Leche League International (LLLI.org), and the American Academy of Pediatrics (HealthyChildren.org). Remember, you don't have to take on doing research and provide links to articles for them. *Point them in the right direction by giving them resources for trustworthy websites and let them do the reading.*

## Week #2

Weekly Goal #1: Breastfeeding a Toddler—If you continue breastfeeding, you don't necessarily need to introduce cow's milk. Human milk is always the better option for your baby. This gets confusing for some families because if a baby was getting formula, then at one year the AAP recommends switching to cow's milk (or a milk alternative), but *if you're breastfeeding, breastmilk is always the recommended option.*

Weekly Goal #2: Handling Criticism—Quoting an authority figure like your pediatrician, the AAP, or the WHO will go a long way toward convincing some people that breastfeeding your toddler is good for them. *Remind well-meaning friends and family that you're all on the same side and want what's best for your child, and the American Academy of Pediatrics recommends continued breastfeeding as long as mutually desired by mom and baby.*

Milestone: The Demand—At 12 months, you should be providing solids at three meals and two snacks each day. However, breastmilk is *still* providing most of the calories and nutrition a baby receives at this age.

## Week #3

**Weekly Goal #1: Breastfeeding a Toddler**—Remember that breastfeeding is more than nutrition to your baby. Your baby may come to you to breastfeed because they are tired, sad, scared, or need a check-in with you. *Be aware that you're meeting your child's emotional needs with breastfeeding and be responsive to those needs.* You might see the check-in feeds increase in frequency if your child is sick or learning a new skill. Be willing to be flexible and deviate from your schedule.

**Weekly Goal #2: Handling Criticism**—*Another option is to not participate in conversations about your feeding choices.* Your baby, your choice. Change the subject when it comes up or let people know the topic is not up for debate and you'd rather not talk about it.

---

**KEY ADVICE: MYTH BUSTER**

*"Breastmilk has no nutrition after the first year." Nope! Breastmilk continues to provide important nutrition and immune factors beyond the first year.* **Breastmilk is beneficial to your child as long as you are able to provide it.**

---

## BREASTFEEDING IN PUBLIC

In many ways, breastfeeding in public becomes even trickier with an older baby. They've now reached the "self-serve" portion of the program and they may pop off unexpectedly, leaving you exposed to onlookers.

Keep in mind that breastfeeding meets the physical and emotional needs of your baby. A breastfeed can be about hunger, a check-in, first aid for an injury, or the snuggle needed to fall asleep.

Here are a couple of things to keep in mind when breastfeeding your older baby. **You are allowed to set limits with your child.** Are you in a place where you'd rather not feed? That's okay; they can wait. Or they can come with you to a place you prefer. **In *all fifty states* of the United States, you have the right to breastfeed your baby anywhere you're allowed to be** (which, by the way, just became legal in 2018, but let's not go there). **You are feeding your baby. Period.** No one has the right to shame or harass you.

Remember, *every time* you breastfeed in public, you are helping normalize public breastfeeding for the moms and babies who will come after you. Feed your baby anywhere, anytime, any *way* that feels most comfortable for you.

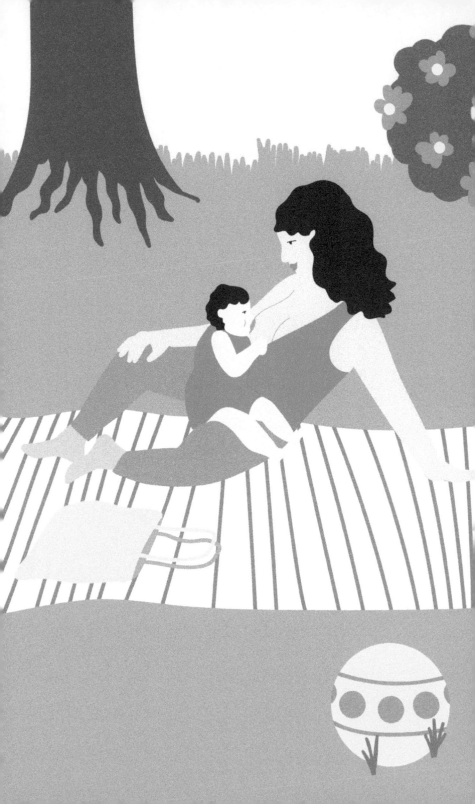

# PART FOUR

# Deciding What's Next

## Breastfeeding Beyond 12 Months

Many families choose to continue offering breastmilk beyond 12 months. Although breastfeeding until age two and beyond is the norm in many other countries, in the Unites States many moms feel a stigma associated with breastfeeding beyond a year. In fact, many refer to feeding beyond a year as "extended breastfeeding," implying that one year was the "normal" time to stop. Remember, though, that the AAP recommends that breastfeeding continue as long as mom and baby find it beneficial.

This chapter offers information on the benefits of breastfeeding your toddler, suggests tips for a successful feeding routine, and discusses pumping for continued bottle-feeding.

## Benefits of Toddler Breastfeeding

Just because a baby is now older than one year doesn't mean breastmilk loses its value. We know, in fact, that breastfeeding beyond a year offers significant benefits.

Even in toddlerhood, breastmilk continues to be an important source of nutrition that supports brain growth.

In the second year of baby's life, 15 ounces of breastmilk provides:

- 29% of energy requirements
- 43% of protein requirements
- 36% of calcium requirements
- 75% of vitamin A requirements
- 76% of folate requirements
- 94% of vitamin B12 requirements
- 60% of vitamin C requirements

Breastmilk also contains immune factors that contribute to fewer illnesses. The American Academy of Family Physicians (AAFP) says that children weaned before two years of age are at increased risk of illness. Along with WHO, they also state that breastfeeding should "ideally continue beyond infancy." But AAFP acknowledges that this is not the cultural norm in the United States despite their assertion that "a natural weaning age for humans is between two and seven years." For this reason, parents who are continuing to breastfeed or are thinking about it require ongoing support and encouragement. For many families, this looks like finding family physicians and pediatricians who understand and are knowledgeable about the ongoing benefits of extended breastfeeding such as "continued immune protection, better social adjustment, and availability of having a sustainable food source in times of emergency." For moms, the longer they breastfeed, the more they decrease their risk of breast cancer.

Don't forget that breastmilk uniquely changes over time and continues to serve the needs of children as they grow older. Research has found that moms who have been lactating for more than one year produce breastmilk that has significantly higher fat and energy contents.

In addition to nutritional benefits, breastfeeding the toddler provides emotional support—soothing frustrations, taming tantrums, and fostering independence and confidence.

## Five Tips for Toddler Breastfeeding

Breastfeeding a toddler is very different than breastfeeding a small baby. Your toddler now has opinions of their own. They are bigger, more energetic, and less likely to sit still during feedings. You will need to have firmer boundaries, and certain breastfeeding situations may require a little more planning.

Let's look at some specific tips for breastfeeding toddlers.

### OFFER A DISTRACTION

Your toddler may decide to feed at an inopportune time for you. Be ready to offer a distraction. If you are in public and you prefer not to breastfeed at that very moment, try offering another snack. Maybe you're in the middle of preparing a meal or trying to get a task done. Try offering a fun activity like stacking food storage containers or playing drums with a pot and a wooden spoon.

Toddlers are also easily distracted by music and games. Put on their favorite song or encourage a funny dance. Pretty soon they will forget they were asking for a breastfeed.

### BE FIRM AND COMMUNICATE

You're in charge and you get to set the rules around feeding. Your child is old enough to understand when you say things like, "We don't feed in bed," or, "We only feed when the sun is out." Once you establish a rule, stick to it so your child knows you aren't going to change your mind. Make breastfeeding work for you.

### DON'T BE AFRAID TO STOP FEEDING

Know when it's time to bring breastfeeding or pumping to an end. Are you dreading breastfeeding? Is it a chore? Do you feel like it's negatively impacting your relationship with your child? It may be time to wrap it up. We previously said never quit on a bad day. But if you've been feeling this way for a while, it may be time to wean or reduce the amount of breastfeeding you're doing, and that's totally okay.

### KNOW WHEN AND WHERE TO BREASTFEED

Where and when to breastfeed is completely up to you. You shouldn't be shamed or made to feel uncomfortable for feeding your baby. Unfortunately, you may get looks from strangers. If you're comfortable breastfeeding your toddler in public, feel good knowing that each time you breastfeed your toddler in public it's an act of "lactivism," helping pave the way for breastfeeding moms who will come after you.

On the other hand, you get to choose when and where. If you're *not* comfortable, your toddler can wait or be offered another source of food. They are no longer at the stage where it can't wait.

## TEACH PROPER CUES

Is your baby using a word for breastfeeding you don't like? Or in the habit of lifting up your shirt in public?

Use this as an opportunity to create rules around breastfeeding and communicate them clearly to your child. You may start using a different word or teach your child to ask instead of lifting up your shirt. What bothers one mom may not bother another. This is all about your comfort zone and adapting to how you want feeding to look as your child gets older.

# Toddler Breastfeeding Schedule

Breastfeeding a toddler is nothing like breastfeeding your young baby. They are active and on the go. Feeds are usually really fast! They are super efficient, experienced breastfeeders now.

Your child may snack frequently or they may want to settle in, get cozy, and nurse for a while as they fall asleep.

You'll probably notice they want to feed when they fall and get hurt or because they are teething and their gums hurt. In a nutshell, every day can be different. So just like life with your toddler, expect the unexpected.

How often should you breastfeed? There's no set number. Some toddlers will nurse one to two times daily and continue doing that for months. Others will breastfeed frequently throughout the day. There's no right or wrong. Make the schedule work for you. Having said that, a typical feeding schedule for a toddler might look something like this:

| 7 a.m. | Wake and breastfeed |
|---|---|
| 8 a.m. | Breakfast (solids) |
| 10 a.m. | Breastfeed and snack (solids) |
| 12 p.m. | Lunch (solids) |
| 3 p.m. | Breastfeed |
| 4 p.m. | Snack (solids) |
| 6 p.m. | Dinner (solids) |
| 7:30 p.m. | Breastfeed before bedtime |

If you're worried your toddler isn't getting enough calories, schedule an appointment with your pediatrician to get a weight check and talk about their nutrition.

## Keep on Pumping

Some moms choose to wrap up feeding at the breast but continue to pump so they can provide breastmilk in a bottle or sippy cup. That may involve pumping once a day or several times a day. The important thing is that you don't make a dramatic change to your feeding or pumping schedule overnight. You want to transition out of one plan and into another (see "Weaning" on page 156).

Your breastmilk supply will adjust to whatever amount of milk removal you are doing. Many moms pump once a day so they can collect a few ounces and give a daily breastmilk snack.

If you think you'll be storing breastmilk for longer than six months, look into a deep freezer. If you end up with extra breastmilk, you can always donate it to another family.

# WILL BREASTFEEDING CAUSE ATTACHMENT ISSUES?

It's a common myth that breastfeeding a child beyond a year creates a dependent child who doesn't become their own person. In fact, moms will tell you the opposite is true. Their breastfed children are independent, curious, and confident. Their children use breastfeeding to calibrate their intense emotions, take a break, and do quick check-ins throughout the day. Breastfeeds tend to be super quick, then the child happily returns to what they were doing.

Experts in the field confirm that breastfeeding beyond a year helps a child grow to be more independent and secure. Elizabeth N. Baldwin, Esq., in "Extended Breastfeeding and the Law" says, "Meeting a child's dependency needs is the key to helping that child achieve independence. And children outgrow these needs according to their own unique timetable." Don't worry, they won't breastfeed forever! There will be a time when they are ready to wrap it up.

So how long is too long? Is there any point at which it's harmful to the child? The AAP states, "There is no upper limit to the duration of breastfeeding and no evidence of psychologic or developmental harm from breastfeeding into the third year of life or longer."

Research by Katherine A. Dettwyler, Ph.D., found that children are actually meant to breastfeed for 2.5 to 7 years. You are *never* harming your child, physically or emotionally, by continuing to breastfeed them. You will know when it's the right time to wean. Follow your gut!

# Weaning

So, it's time to wrap up breastfeeding. Congratulations, you did it! Whether you met your goal or you wish your breastfeeding journey had been different, feel good about what you accomplished. There's no room for judgment, guilt, or shame. You are making the decision that's best for your family.

If you're having mixed feelings, you're not alone. It's normal to experience conflicting emotions at this stage. Sometimes you're the one who is ready to wean, sometimes the child initiates weaning, and sometimes weaning happens naturally. Moms often describe weaning as bittersweet. It's the end of a special part of your relationship with your child.

This chapter offers information on the emotional impact of weaning, night weaning, and baby-led weaning as well as knowing when it's time to wean and how to introduce solids.

## How Weaning Will Affect You

There's a good chance you have conflicting feelings about weaning. Even if you're 100 percent sure it is the right decision, you might still be a little sad. Any feelings you're having are valid. For many reasons, weaning is often emotional. You'll also experience fluctuating hormones as you wean (just like at the beginning of pregnancy) that may intensify your feelings.

Many moms find it helpful to mark the end of breastfeeding with something meaningful. You might write a letter to your child about what breastfeeding meant to the two of you, celebrate with a dinner out, take a picture of the last breastfeed, write a note on the last bag of frozen milk, buy something for yourself, or tell the world on social media you're done.

Be on the look out for how weaning affects your mental health. Weaning can trigger postpartum depression or postpartum anxiety in some moms. If you are concerned you are experiencing either of those, reach out to a therapist, your doctor, or check out Postpartum Support International at 1-800-944-4773 for help in English or Spanish or go to Postpartum.net.

## Signs It's Time to Wean

Some moms are completely certain the time is right to wean, whereas others have shifting feelings from day to day. Look at it like a scale. If in your decision-making process on whether to wean, the no-to-breastfeeding side has stayed down for a while (even though you may see the yes/no scale go back and forth), it may be the right time. If you're still unsure, try sitting with the decision for a week and see how it feels.

On the other hand, sometimes your child is the one who makes the decision. That can be tough if you're not ready. Or welcome, if you're both in the same place.

Either way, remember: Weaning *isn't quitting*; you're just moving on to the next stage.

## WEANING AT SIX MONTHS

Six months is a common time for some moms to wean. You've started introducing solids, and your baby is getting much more active. When you wean before a year, you'll be replacing breastmilk with formula. If possible, try to stretch out the remaining breastmilk so your baby gets less and less each day as you transition formula in.

Solids and formula can both be constipating, so you may want to keep a food log and pay attention to how formula and solids are affecting your baby and how often they are stooling. If you notice stooling slowing down, avoid those foods that are having a constipating effect. You can bring them back later when your child can tolerate them better.

If your baby is constipated, try offering more fruit juice (prune or pear) or foods that will help move stools (see "Constipation" on page 116). If you notice that your baby hasn't stooled in a couple of days and they seem uncomfortable, try using your hand to massage their tummy in a circular motion. This works great after a bath when they are already relaxed.

## WEANING AT 12 MONTHS

Weaning at one year means your child won't need formula. Rather, you'll substitute cow's milk or an alternative milk for breastmilk as you wean.

You may also see a sharp decline in how hungry your child is at 12 months. Baby is probably less interested in eating or may reject foods they previously loved. This is all super normal. Take some comfort in knowing their growth rate slows pretty dramatically at this age so they don't need as many calories as they previously did (about 1,000 calories each day from their three meals and two snacks).

# Night-Weaning

Many moms decide to start off by weaning their babies from nighttime feeds first, then gradually wean them altogether.

Night-weaning is different for each child. Some adjust fairly easily if you create a new feeding routine and stick to it, whereas others might push back on the new plan. If you are co-sleeping or bed sharing, you may need to change rooms for a few nights and have your partner take over nighttime care. This requires some planning to pick the right time so it works for you as a couple.

A few things to keep in mind when you night-wean:

+ Make sure your child is still gaining weight appropriately.

+ They will feed more frequently during the day to make up the calories. Be responsive to their feeding cues.

+ They may want more physical connection during the day as they adjust to the dropped nighttime feeds. Bring them in for lots of cuddles!

## Solids and Your Toddler

As your toddler gets older, nudge them toward foods that are increasingly more complex in texture and flavor. A common technique is to offer them a favorite food alongside a new food. You may be able to start to give them many of the same foods you're having for your meal, which makes mealtime so much easier. Just watch heavily spiced, salted, or sweetened foods, and make sure the texture is appropriate.

One-year-olds are known for being picky eaters. If your little one is developing picky eating habits:

* Keep offering the food they rejected. It can take 10 times or more of being offered a food before children decide whether they like it.

* Eat together. Seeing what you eat has a powerful influence on your child.

* Make it fun. Try involving your toddler in meals by letting them choose foods or help in the preparation. And remember to keep mealtimes stress-free. It's better for everyone.

As you introduce foods, don't restrict fats. Toddlers get about half their calories from fat, which is essential to their growth and nutrition right now.

Safety warning: Continue to observe your toddler at meals. Don't leave them unattended. You should be watching for choking and that they remain safely seated.

## BABY-LED WEANING

Baby-led weaning is a technique, beginning around six months, that lets the baby control what and how much they eat by feeding themselves. Babies start with finger-foods, not purees or baby food. Parents do not spoon-feed babies. The parent is in charge of *what* they are offered, when it's offered, and what form it's in. Baby decides what to eat, how much to eat, and how fast to eat.

This can be a really fun, if messy, time for your family. When offering babies solids, make sure to go with large pieces of soft foods cut into wedge shapes that make it easy for baby to gnaw on. Then sit back and watch the show. Seriously, don't intervene if baby starts squishing or smashing the food. This is all a perfectly normal part of the experience. Be patient and don't expect your baby to get it right away. Relax and have fun with it; they'll figure out how to eat. We all do. In the meantime, get all the cute pics and videos you can!

Proponents of baby-led weaning say it fosters a healthier relationship with food, makes feeding time easier and less stressful, and helps prevent obesity later in life. Some medical providers have concerns about a higher risk of choking, but whether that's an issue has not been determined. Parents who use baby-led weaning report that choking is no more of an issue than feeding purees and mashed foods.

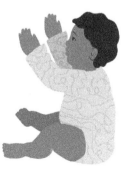

# Conclusion

Well, we've reached the end, and regardless of whether breast-feeding was everything you hoped it would be, take a moment to look back on everything you accomplished. Feel proud knowing you worked hard and you breastfed your baby. You did a GREAT job!

I hope you've found this book helpful and that the information and tips provided improved your breastfeeding experience.

Enjoy your little one and all the wonderful stages that are yet to come on your parenting journey!

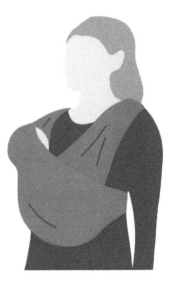

# Resources

## BOOKS

*The Breastfeeding Book* by Martha Sears and William Sears

*Breastfeeding Made Simple* by Nancy Mohrbacher and Kathleen Tendall-Tackett

*Ina May's Guide to Breastfeeding* by Ina May Gaskin

*Lactivate! A User's Guide to Breastfeeding* by Jill Krause and Chrisie Rosenthal

*Life with Baby Workbook* by Amy Tucker and Erin Fassnacht

*The Nursing Mother's Companion* and *The Nursing Mother's Guide to Weaning* by Kathleen Huggins

*The Womanly Art of Breastfeeding* by La Leche League International

## WEBSITES

**American Academy of Pediatrics**
HealthyChildren.org/English/ages-stages/baby/breastfeeding

**Breastfeeding after Breast and Nipple Surgeries**
BFAR.org/index.shtml

**KellyMom** (evidence-based breastfeeding information)
KellyMom.com

**La Leche League USA** or **La Leche League International**
LLLUSA.org or LLLI.org

**The Land of Milk and Mommy** (virtual lactation consultations and resources)
LandOfMilkAndMommy.com

**Nancy Mohrbacher** (reliable breastfeeding information)
NancyMohrbacher.com

**Dr. Jack Newman** (great videos and fact sheets from one of the leading experts in breastfeeding)
IBCOnline.ca

**Postpartum Support International**
1-800-944-4473 or Postpartum.net

**Dr. Sears** (respected pediatrician and breastfeeding expert)
AskDrSears.com/topics/feeding-eating/breastfeeding

## SUPPORT GROUPS

Places to look for support groups near you:

+ Breastfeeding stores
+ Hospitals
+ Lactation Consultant offices
+ La Leche League

# References

Akobeng, A. K., A. V. Ramanan, I. Buchan, and R. F. Heller. "Effect of Breast Feeding on Risk of Coeliac Disease: A Systematic Review and Meta-Analysis of Observational Studies." *Archives of Disease in Childhood* 91, no. 1 (May 10, 2005): 39–43, doi: 10.1136 /adc.2005.082016.

American Academy of Family Physicians. "Breastfeeding, Family Physicians Supporting (Position Paper)." Accessed July 14, 2020, aafp.org/about/policies/all/breastfeeding-support.html.

American Academy of Pediatrics. "Benefits of Breastfeeding for Mom." Last updated July 25, 2016, healthychildren.org/English /ages-stages/baby/breastfeeding/Pages/Benefits-of-Breastfeeding -for-Mom.aspx.

———. "Breastfeeding Benefits Your Baby's Immune System." Last updated August 8, 2016, healthychildren.org/English /ages-stages/baby/breastfeeding/Pages/Breastfeeding -Benefits-Your-Babys-Immune-System.aspx.

———. "Breastfeeding Policy Statement: Breastfeeding and the Use of Human Milk" *Pediatrics* 115, no. 2 (Feb. 2005): 496–506, pediatrics.aappublications.org/content/115/2/496.

———. "Constipation in Children." Last updated February 28, 2017, healthychildren.org/English/health-issues/conditions /abdominal/Pages/Constipation.aspx.

———. "Teething: 4 to 7 Months." Last updated October 6, 2016, healthychildren.org/English/ages-stages/baby/teething -tooth-care/Pages/Teething-4-to-7-Months.aspx.

———. "Where We Stand: Breastfeeding." Last updated July 11, 2014, healthychildren.org/English/ages-stages/baby /breastfeeding/Pages/Where-We-Stand-Breastfeeding.aspx.

Baldwin, Elizabeth. "Extended Breastfeeding and the Law." *Breastfeeding Abstracts* 20, no. 3 (February 2001): 19–20, singlemomontherun.com/2012/05/27/extended -breastfeeding-and-the-law.

Barclay, Andrew R., Richard K. Russell, Michelle L. Wilson, W. Harper Gilmour, Jack Satsangi, and David C. Wilson. "Systematic Review: The Role of Breastfeeding in the Development of Pediatric Inflammatory Bowel Disease." *The Journal of Pediatrics* 155, no. 3 (September 2009): 421–26, doi: 10.1016/j.jpeds.2009.03.017.

Barros, Fernando C., Cesar G. Victora, Tereza Cristina Semer, Santos Tonioli Filho, Elaine Tomasi, and Elisabete Weiderpass. "Use of Pacifiers Is Associated with Decreased Breast-Feeding Duration." *Pediatrics* 95, no. 4 (April 1995): 497–99, pediatrics .aappublications.org/content/95/4/497.

Bonyata, Kelly. "Do Breastfeeding Mothers Need Extra Calories or Fluids?" KellyMom.com. Last updated March 19, 2019, kellymom .com/nutrition/mothers-diet/mom-calories-fluids.

———. "How Does a Mother's Diet Affect Her Milk?" KellyMom .com. Last updated January 14, 2018, kellymom.com/nutrition /mothers-diet/mom-diet.

———. "How Much Expressed Milk Will My Baby Need?" *KellyMom.com.* Accessed July 14, 2020, kellymom.com/bf /pumpingmoms/pumping/milkcalc.

Centers for Disease Control and Prevention. "CDC Releases 2018 Breastfeeding Report Card." Accessed July 14, 2020, cdc.gov/media/releases/2018/p0820-breastfeeding-report-card.html.

Clemens, John, Remon Abu Elyazeed, Malla Rao, MEngg MPH, Stephen Savarino, Badria Z. Morsy, Yongdai Kim, Thomas Wierzba, Abdollah Naficy, and Y. Jack Lee. "Early Initiation of Breastfeeding and the Risk of Infant Diarrhea in Rural Egypt." *Pediatrics* 104, no. 1 (July 1999): e3, doi: 10.1542/peds.104.1.e3.

Cleveland Clinic. "Kangaroo Care." Last updated June 29, 2020, my.clevelandclinic.org/health/treatments/12578 -kangaroo-care.

Cochi, Stephen L., David W. Fleming, Allen W. Hightower, Khanchit Limpakarnjanarat, Richard R. Facklam, J. David Smith, R. Keith Sikes, and Claire V. Broome. "Primary Invasive *Haemophilus Influenzae* Type B Disease: A Population-Based Assessment of Risk Factors." *The Journal of Pediatrics* 108, no. 6 (June 1986): 887–96, doi:10.1016/s0022-3476(86)80922-2.

Doan, Therese, Caryl L. Gay, Holly P. Kennedy, Jack Newman, and Kathryn A. Lee. "Nighttime Breastfeeding Behavior Is Associated with More Nocturnal Sleep among First-Time Mothers at One Month Postpartum." *Journal of Clinical Sleep Medicine* 10, no. 3 (March 15, 2014): 313–19, doi: 10.5664/jcsm.3538.

Ip, Stanley, Mei Chung, Gowri Raman, Thomas A. Trikalinos, and Joseph Lau. "A Summary of the Agency for Healthcare Research and Quality's Evidence Report on Breastfeeding in Developed Countries." *Breastfeeding Medicine* 4, no. s1 (October 14, 2009): S-17-S-30, doi:10.1089/bfm.2009.0050.

Johnson, Melinda. "Breastfeeding Builds a Better Jaw, and Other Benefits for Babies." *U.S. News & World Report.* Accessed July 19, 2020, health.usnews.com/health-news/blogs/eat-run/2014/08/29/breastfeeding-builds-a-better-jaw-and-other-benefits-for-babies.

Jordan, Susan J., Victor Siskind, Adèle C. Green, David C. Whiteman, and Penelope M. Webb. "Breasfeeding and Risk of Epithelial Ovarian Cancer." *Cancer Causes & Control* 21, no. 1 (January 2010): 109–16, jstor.org/stable/25621334?seq=1.

KellyMom.com. "Average Weight Gain for Breastfed Babies." Last updated January 27, 2018, kellymom.com/bf/normal/weight-gain.

———. "Extended Breastfeeding Factsheet." Accessed July 14, 2020, kellymom.com/store/freehandouts/extended_bf_factsheet.pdf.

———. "Healing with Breastmilk." Last updated January 14, 2018, kellymom.com/bf/can-i-breastfeed/illness-surgery/healing-breastmilk.

———. "How Can I Use Breastfeeding to Prevent Pregnancy?" Accessed July 14, 2020, kellymom.com/store/handouts/newborn/LAM.pdf.

———. "Natural Treatments for Nursing Moms." Last updated April 8, 2020, kellymom.com/bf/can-i-breastfeed/herbs/natural-treatments.

La Leche League International. "Colostrum: General." Accessed July 19, 2020, llli.org/breastfeeding-info/colostrum-general.

Liaw, Jen-Jiuan, Luke Yang, Yin Ti, Susan Tucker Blackburn, Yue-Cune Chang, and Liang-Wen Sun. "Non-Nutritive Sucking

Relieves Pain for Preterm Infants during Heel Stick Procedures in Taiwan." *Journal of Clinical Nursing* 19, no. 19–20 (September 15, 2010): 2741–51, doi: 10.1111/j.1365-2702.2010.03300.x.

Mandel, Dror, Ronit Lubetzky, Shaul Dollberg, Shimon Barak, and Francis B. Mimouni. "Fat and Energy Contents of Expressed Human Breast Milk in Prolonged Lactation." *Pediatrics* 116, no. 3 (September 2005): e432–35, doi: 10.1542/peds.2005-0313.

Mannion, Cynthia A., Amy J. Hobbs, Sheila W. McDonald, and Suzanne C. Tough. "Maternal Perceptions of Partner Support during Breastfeeding." *International Breastfeeding Journal* 8, no. 1 (May 8, 2013), doi: 10.1186/1746-4358-8-4.

Milligan Newmark, Lauren. "From Mother's Gut to Milk." International Milk Genomics Consortium. Accessed July 19, 2020, milkgenomics.org/article/from-mothers-gut-to-milk.

Morton, Jane. "Maximizing Milk Production with Hands-On Pumping." *Newborn Nursery at Lucile Packard Children's Hospital, Stanford Medicine.* Accessed July 19, 2020, med.stanford.edu/newborns/professional-education/breastfeeding/maximizing-milk-production.html.

National Institutes of Health. "Calcium." Last modified December 6, 2019, ods.od.nih.gov/factsheets/Calcium-Consumer.

Rapaport, Lisa. "Can Breastfeeding Reduce Babies' Pain During Vaccinations?" *Reuters.* Accessed July 14, 2020, in.reuters.com/article/us-health-babies-vaccine-pain/can-breastfeeding-reduce-babies-pain-during-vaccinations-idINKBN13D29K.

Saarinen, Ulla M., and Merja Kajosaari. "Breastfeeding as Prophylaxis against Atopic Disease: Prospective Follow-Up Study until 17 Years Old." *The Lancet* 346, no. 8982 (October 21, 1995): 1065–69. doi: 10.1016/s0140-6736(95)91742-x.

Stuart-Macadam, Patricia and Katherine A. Dettwyler. *Breastfeeding: Biocultural Perspectives.* New York: Aldine de Gruyter, 1995.

University of Texas Medical Branch at Galveston. "Breastfeeding, Vaccinations Help Reduce Ear Infection Rates in Babies: Lower Smoking Rates Also a Factor." *ScienceDaily.com.* Accessed July 19., 2020, sciencedaily.com/releases/2016/03/160328084906 .htm.

Warren, John J., Steven M. Levy, H. Lester Kirchner, Arthur J. Nowak, George R. Bergus. "Pacifier Use and the Occurrence of Otitis Media in the First Year of Life." *Pediatric Dentistry* 23, no. 2 (February 2001): 103–7, aapd.org/globalassets/media /publications/archives/warren-23-02.pdf.

Wiessinger, Diane, Diana West, Linda J. Smith, and Teresa Pitman. *Sweet Sleep: Nighttime and Naptime Strategies for the Breastfeeding Family.* New York: La Leche League International and Ballantine Books, 2014.

World Health Organization (WHO). "The WHO Child Growth Standards." Accessed July 14, 2020, WHO.int/childgrowth/en.

———. "Maternal, Newborn, Child and Adolescent Health: Breastfeeding." Accessed July 14, 2020, who.int /maternal_child_adolescent/topics/child/nutrition /breastfeeding/en.

# Index

# Acknowledgments

I have been blessed with the love and support of so many, and my gratitude runs deep. My three sons—Ben, Ethan, and Sam—are the reason I pursued this work. I love you so much, sweet boys! You are my heart and my motivation.

Thank you to all my breastfeeding families for inviting me into your lives at a very special and vulnerable time and for sharing your sweet babies.

I'd be lost without my village. Thank you to everyone who encourages me, including my parents Bill and Sharon, my sister Vickie, Saul, Maryssa, Alex, Nancy, Stacy, Barie, Rebecca, Dawn, Cheri, Cathie, Tara, Andrea, Rani, Bekah, Caitlyn, Molly, Inna, Jessamyn, Jenny, Barb, Carly Bev, Callie, Briana, Kirsty, and everyone at Cleo.

Thank you to my mentors, Gini Baker and Karen Hatcher, and to my students who taught me as I taught them: Carrie, Amelia, Devorie, Inna, Nikki, and Sarah.

# About the Author

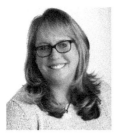

Chrisie Rosenthal is a highly respected IBCLC in Los Angeles and mom to three teenage boys, two dogs, and two guinea pigs. She studied lactation and perinatal education at UCSD, became an IBCLC, and founded her private practice, The Land of Milk and Mommy. She has helped thousands of families reach their breastfeeding goals. She provides virtual classes, including Introduction to Breastfeeding, Return-to-Work, and Pumping & Bottle-feeding. She's the co-author of *Lactivate! A User's Guide to Breastfeeding*. You can reach her at LandOfMilkAndMommy.com or on Instagram @thelandofmilkandmommy.